LIVE LONGEST Book 1:

The MISSING KEYS

Identifying the Problems

The Medical Avoidance of Illness and Disability

Dr Mileham Hayes

Publishing Details

Updates

Updated information will be regularly provided free for subscribers on the website: http://livelongest.com.au

Sources

Most of the evidence, data, studies and trials in ***Live Longest*** are accessed from the top medical journals and national statistics after the year 2000. Most are the latest available. National surveys and audits can cover longer time periods; but these older figures and statistics are still relevant. Some graphs used are preferred because they are the most user friendly. This information was up to date as of the end of the financial year 2016.

Lies, Damned Lies And Statistics

This is a book for the general reader. I have tried not to saturate it with too many overwhelming and boring figures; but the references are there for the medical reader or anyone who wants more detail. Where and when the study is so huge it should convince even the greatest skeptic, I may give a number or a percentage that is relevant and reassuring—such as the finding that meditation reduced cardiovascular events by 45%, which even encouraged me to try it.

Disclaimer

This book is for information only and should not be used for any treatment without consulting and discussing it with your doctor. Opinions and techniques differ within the medical profession. The author and publisher expressly disclaim responsibility for any consequence arising from use of the information in this book.

First published as HELP – Health Extension Life Programs (2007). Second edition completely revised and updated to July 2016.
Third edition revised and updated 2017.

ISBN: 9780995399617 (pbk)

PREFACE

When I was appointed to the world's first Coronary Care Unit we revolutionized the treatment of heart attacks and it was expected that throughout the Western World we would soon not only treat, but also prevent this, our greatest killer, cardiovascular disease.

However, 50 years later, after men have gone to the moon, color TV, the Internet, Facebook, Computers, Smart Phones and Watches and absolutely incredible similar advances in medicine, the American College of Cardiology 65th Annual Scientific Session in 2016 reported, *"Analysis of (the last) two decades reveal risk factors are on the rise...Despite increased understanding of heart disease risk factors and the need for preventive lifestyle changes, patients are suffering the most severe type at a younger age, and they are more likely to have preventable risk factors".*

I'll run that by you again: "*They are <u>more likely</u> to have <u>preventable risk factors</u>*" (and they are younger).

And this goes for all the other illnesses that can kill us earlier than the lifespan we should live.

The next greatest illness that cuts us down in our prime or, at least many years before we should die, is cancer of the colon. And this too keeps increasing.

The third greatest killer is lung cancer and here, at last, some improvement has been made due to the reduction in cigarette smoking, which, incidentally, my father ceased three years before the world no-smoking campaign. He was ahead of his time in many aspects of preventive medicine, which is how and why he practised until he was 84 years old.

We are now living in a toxic environment whare processed food in available 24 hours a day, seven days a week. Labour saving devices reduce what used to be normal daily activity. Television, computers and smart phones encourage further sedentary behavior. The Diseases of

Affluence, (obesity, cardiovascular disease, high cholesterol, hypertension, depression, diabetes) are epidemic. We are working longer, harder and are more stressed.

But, be that as it may, heart attacks, most cancers and, in fact, most of the illnesses that cut us down before our full lifespan *can be prevented.*

The first thing to do is "know your enemy", to know *exactly* what illness is waiting to get you, now, at your present age and to know "*the preventable risk factors"* and how to predict and avoid these conditions.

But most of us, including my medical colleagues, don't know exactly what illnesses occur, in what order, for our age.

These are The MISSING KEYS.

If we knew them, *and now we can,* we could take specific avoiding preventive measures.

This then is B**OOK 1 of LIVE LONGEST - The MISSING KEYS.**

The other books in this series form a continuum covering all aspects to LIVE LONGER HEALTHIER.

Dr Mileham Hayes OAM, MB,BS (Qld), FRCP (Edin), FRCP (Lon)

The MISSING KEYS *are those illnesses, behaviors, conditions or accidents, which cause our early premature death or disablement.*

No one dies early from "natural causes" but, because this information has only recently become available, these formerly **Missing Keys** had not been identified, let alone utilized, to predict and therefore head-off, these health problems that cause our premature demise or disabilities.

Now official National Lists order and prioritize these illnesses for each age group of our lives.

"Death from old age is inevitable but death before old age is not" and if we can now identify the illnesses, these MISSING KEYS, that we are most likely to encounter, we can use this information to provide the best chances of preventing or avoiding them, being healthy, not prematurely dying or being disabled.

LIVE LONGEST is a series covering all aspects of our health and is the most systematic and logical approach to our health:

1. Identify the illnesses most likely for our age and prevent or avoid them: the **MISSING KEYS**

2. Find out the most beneficial foods that can prevent most illnesses: **NEWTRITION**

3. Learn how to avoid the age declines in capacity and health: **SUCCESSFUL AGING**

4. Be informed as to the best **EXERCISE** for your age and attain the **OPTIMUM WEIGHT**

5. The **"Big 11"** - practical information on Specific Illnesses

6. **Other Health Issues**: Not necessarily illnesses.

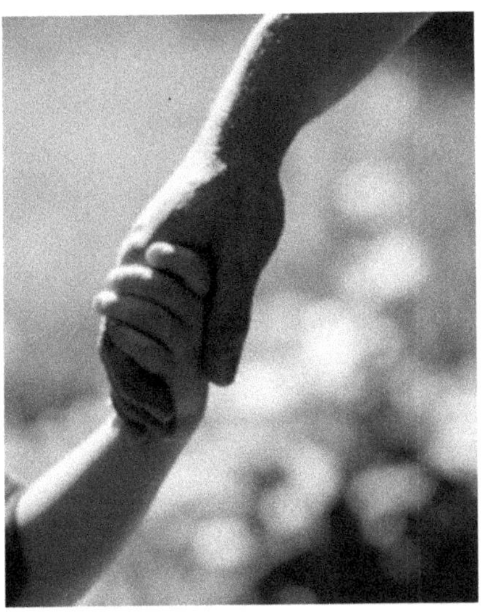

Live Longest Series
Books for Total Health and Longevity

Book 1: **The Missing Keys:** *The Medical Avoidance of Illness and Disability*

Book 2: **Newtrition:** *The most complete, evidenced foods to prevent illnesses*

Book 3: **Successful Aging-Optimum Health**: *The Quality of Life and Death*

Other Titles

- Exercise and Activity
- Optimum Weight
- Specific Illnesses
    - **Expands on specific illnesses with information and practical advice not usually covered or known**
      Heart Attacks, Atrial Fibrillation, Hypertension, Stroke, Cancer, Alzheimer's, Osteoporosis, Osteoarthritis, Low Back Pain, Coeliac Disease, Diabetes
- Specific Issues:
    - **Expands on specific issues, not necessarily illnesses, again with information not usually covered or known**
      Women's and Men's Issues, Skin, Hygiene, Head To Toes, Complementary and Alternative Medicine (CAM), Happiness, Stress, Meditation, Depression - Psychiatry, Sleep

Simple, definitive, gentle plans and core programs medically proven to work.

http: //livelongest.com.au

Definitions

Health

"A state of complete physical, mental and social wellbeing and not merely the absence of disease or infirmity." —World Health Organization, 1946

Quality of Life (QOL)

This is a relatively new concept and there is a lack of agreement, with over a hundred definitions. As society becomes more complex, so do expectations, and hence the criteria increase. It is important to consider the broader concerns of the individual. This is a changing concept that takes into account the general well-being of individuals and societies, outlining negative and positive features of life, and observing life satisfaction, including physical health, family, education, employment, wealth, religious beliefs, finance and the environment.

Live Longest

Optimization of present health and fitness: to minimize any illnesses and disabilities; to stay mentally alert, active, healthy, independent and socially integrated, with the capacity to cope with change; for the whole of our predicted lifespan with respect to personal, social, spiritual, emotional and economic goals and restrictions.

While this is a mouthful, it covers all areas and contingencies, many of which we don't consider when we are young—such as being able to remain independent with enough money to do so.

Cost-Effectiveness

"Health improvement gained dollar for dollar."

Research into cost-effectiveness in preventive medicine found "the appropriate criterion is not cost savings but acceptable value for money."[1] "Acceptable" meant "a health improvement outcome" and it was found that "Americans were willing to spend money to get better health outcomes."

Cost Beneficial

Major illnesses involve an unmeasurable amount of disruption, both emotionally and financially, to the patient, family and employer. It may well thus be more beneficial, but not as cost-effective, to the patient to pay more to minimize these downstream effects if possible.

Compression of Morbidity

The postponement of disabling conditions without necessarily extending life itself.

Focus

The most cost-effective optimization of present and future health. In effect this means concentrating on those illnesses that can be prevented or cured.

Preventive Medicine

The cost-effective prevention or early diagnosis of illness by evidence-based criteria to maximize health, longevity, independence and minimize disabilities.

Disability

The World Health Organization defines disability as an umbrella term that encompasses impairments, activity limitations and participation restrictions that reflect the complex interaction between "features of a person's body and features of the society in which he or she lives." The Americans With Disabilities Act tells us that disability is "a physical or mental impairment that substantially limits one or more major life activities."

All nations have their own specific definitions such as any of the following limitations, restrictions or impairments that have lasted or are likely to last > 6 months (1998 Australian Bureau Statistics):

- Loss of sight, hearing, speech not corrected by glasses/aids
- Chest pain, shortness of breath, nervous condition, brain injury or any other long-term condition that restricts everyday activity
- Blackouts, fits - Difficulty learning
- Incomplete use of arms, fingers, legs, feet. Difficulty gripping.
- Restriction in physical activities or work - Disfigurement or deformity
- Mental condition that needs help or supervision
- Treatment medication for long-term condition

High-/Low-Density Food: High or low calorie content

Nutrient-Rich/Poor: Good and beneficial food or poor-quality junk and pap.

The ideal food is low-density, nutrient-rich.

What This Book Offers – The Missing Keys

There are many excellent books on good health practices (and very many bad ones), but to date none seem to have identified which specific illnesses are most likely to disable or kill you at your present age.

These books, no matter how good, tell only half the story; avoiding or minimizing illness is the other half. There are no books I have found that cover all aspects of staying healthy with a good quality of life (QOL). Most books ignore the handicaps that illnesses can impose.

Advances and new discoveries in medicine make some topics hot favorites. The latest foci of interest are the gut microbiome (the micro-organisms inhabiting our gastrointestinal tract) and inflammation. While there may be truth to certain aspects of these conditions, the narrow focus does not account for high-risk behaviors and lifestyle factors responsible for many premature and avoidable deaths.

Our genes only account for 25% of our longevity. In other words 75% is up to you—and up to you now!

Prevention should focus on what illness is most likely for you now, at your age, this year... and how to avoid it. Predictive analysis investigates this question with official decade-by-decade lists of causes of death and disabilities. Age and gender-relevant tests and investigations are then detailed to enable you to avoid or diagnose them early enough to cure.

This approach provides the most essential information, **"The Missing Keys,"** for how to live longest and avoid the target illnesses.

Past Failures – Present Advances

Free health programs and free health services have not cut premature deaths or kept people out of hospitals anywhere in the First World. These programs include the United States' "most intensive and expensive trial ever"—the US$180 million MRFIT program free to volunteers[2]—and the United Kingdom's National Health Scheme (their recent "MoT" program), and 15 international health-screening programs. Nor have the annual routine check-ups where 44 million Americans a year "derived no benefit from their annual physical."[3] Such efforts have all been an incredible waste of money, false hopes, false promises and "overwhelming failures."

In fact even with completely free hospitals and treatments in the United Kingdom the health of the lower socioeconomic classes has got progressively three times worse, whereas rich people are living longer.

Why and How Do People Live Longer?

Why do some people live longer? Of course genetics plays a part, but, as already pointed out, it is estimated that 75% of premature aging is due to environmental and lifestyle factors. While the rich live longer, most of the longest-living groups, in the so-called Blue Zones, are poor peasant societies. By combining the lifestyles of these Blue Zones with the expensive advanced medical treatments that the rich enjoy, it is obvious that the chances of living longer and healthier are maximized.

There has been, however, one other factor not previously identified or highlighted which has, until now, been the "Missing Keys" and is a key revelation of this book.

The Missing Keys and Age-Specific Prevention

The unique contribution of ***Live Longest Missing Keys*** is that it provides Age-Specific Predictive Analysis. This information has only recently become available and is based on international official government data which lists, in order, the illnesses most likely to cause death or disabilities for each age group and sex.

Death from old age is inevitable, but premature deaths are mostly avoidable tragedies. If you and your doctor don't know what illnesses you are most likely to encounter at your age that cause these premature deaths or disabilities, how can the correct preventive measures be instituted? Yet many doctors don't consult or know these lists.

Knowing these lists are the **"Missing Keys"** that allows for the most complete health plan to optimize longer life.

Specific identification and focus now allows for the prevention of the illnesses which are most likely to kill or disable you this year—and every other year, for that matter.

These lists are now made available in age and sex dedicated chapters. In addition, complete health plans and programs are detailed for your age *now*, as a substitute for the "one size fits all" annual physical.

"Someone told me that each equation I included in the book would halve the sales".

Stephen Hawking "A Brief History of Time" 1988

That said:

One of my daughters said "there are too many graphs" which was the stimulus for me to re-jig and update this 3rd Edition wherein I have merged as many graphs as I can while dedicating single chapters exclusive to the age and sex of you, the reader, so you don't have to read any others.

So, for those intrepid readers who press on, I do apologize for the tables and graphs but they do best explain things at a glance...(and sales are great...thankyou).

MGH 2017

Abbreviations

BMJ – British Medical Journal

JAMA – Journal of the American Medical Association

NEJM – New England Journal of Medicine

BG – Blood Glucose

BP – Blood Pressure

CAC – Cancer of the Colon

CAD – Coronary Artery Disease

CDC – Centers for Disease Control and Prevention

CVS – Cardiovascular System

CLRTD - Chronic Lower Respiratory Disease

COPD – Chronic Obstructive Pulmonary Disease (Asthma, Emphysema, Interstitial Fibrosis)

ECG/EKG - Electrocardiogram

FDA – Federal Drug Administration

H/L DL – High- or Low-Density Cholesterol

HT – Hypertension – raised BP

IHD – Ischemic Heart Disease – essentially the same as CAD

MVA/RTA – Motor Vehicle/Road Traffic Accidents

Terminology

Terminology differs and duplicates. Ischemic Heart Disease (IHD) and Coronary Artery Disease (CAD) are effectively synonymous. What the United States calls a "stroke" other countries may include under cerebrovascular disease. Emphysema, asthma and bronchitis can be covered by Chronic Obstructive Pulmonary Disease (COPD)

Experience and Evidence:

Live Longest is based on a series of lectures and seminars the author first presented at the University of Queensland in 2007. Now a series of books, ***Live Longest*** covers most aspects of our current health issues. This first book, ***The Missing Keys***, now in its *3rd Edition,* uniquely identifies the illnesses pertinent to our age and sex and how to avoid or prevent them. Because of the size to cover the whole health spectrum, it has necessitated a series of books. It is recommended the reader accesses the full details in these sequel books. Also available will be regular free updates on Facebook.

Author Profile

Mileham studied medicine at the University of Queensland and became the first graduate selected to a Sydney Teaching Hospital where he was appointed to the world's first Coronary Care Unit as well as running one of the earliest Sports Clinics. He volunteered for the Viet Nam War and was seconded to the Main Military Hospital.

Specialist studies in both Edinburgh and London saw him elevated to being a Fellow of both Royal Colleges of Physicians. He studied in one of the foundation Obesity Units and did research into STDs and Vitamin C. He even learned acupuncture from the first doctor to bring it out of China (Felix Mann of London). On returning to Australia he practised as a GP/PCP, concentrating on prevention, then as a forensic specialist, and now in his preventive medicine and skin cancer clinic. He is the author of two medical texts: *Skin Cancer, Melanoma and Mimics* and *Practical Skin Cancer Surgery* (Elsevier, Churchill-Livingstone).

This book was originally intended as another medical text but the information is so beneficial for anyone interested in optimizing and maximizing their own health it has been rewritten it for a general audience.

Preventive medicine is Mileham's passion, stimulated by his father who was also a clinician and practiced until he was 84 years old, passing on his shrewd, now proven, observations. Such common sense and age-old wisdom is also incorporated in this book along with the basis of evidence. Preventive Medicine is, at last, undergoing a revolution in research, with advances seemingly made each week, if not each day.

On a personal note, he put himself through medicine by farming and playing jazz, played most sports at a high level (rugby, cricket, tennis), was an inveterate surfer, and drove fast enough for BP to offer him sponsorship. As an Air Force reservist he had many adventures including flying with the CIA and being "interviewed" by the Marshal of the Royal Air Force. As an internationally touring musician he had his own ABC radio and national TV shows and ran award-winning jazz and blues festivals. He was a regular columnist for three leading newspapers and a medical journal. He was awarded the Order of Australia in 1991. A passionate gardener, cook and lover of art and literature, in spare moments he writes bad poetry and good limericks. He is in full-time private practice, is married with five children, has five grandchildren and lives in the country, where his wife breeds award-winning cattle and chocolate Labradors.

How This Book Was Written: "Funny Times and Common Sense".

When I was a medical student I was fortunate to be mentored by one of the world's greatest surgeons, Sir Clarence Legget. I was arguably the worst student because I was in a very successful jazz band and had appeared and played with some of the world's greatest legends. I also played cricket, rugby, and tennis, surfed and liked girls a lot, all of which didn't leave much time for studying. But "Clarrie" taught, or refined in me, clinical acumen.

He would pause with us eight or so students at the door of the ward and ask us, "Who should we see first?" and "What is your diagnosis?"

The rest of my group, diligent little sots, knew much more than I did and trotted out incredible diagnoses. I was last and when Clarrie asked me, I blurted out, "Bed 16."

"And why is that, Mileham?" Clarrie asked.

As I didn't have a clue what was actually wrong with the patient, I further lamely blurted out, "Because she looks the sickest."

A now very agitated Sir Clarence exclaimed, "Yes, yes, yes!" and turned on the rest of my group saying, "Why can't you be like Mileham! She is obviously the sickest and it is she who demands our priority attention. Class dismissed!" I was not very popular with my group after that.

Fast-forward five years and I was attached to the doyen of Scottish Medicine, Sir Hugh Munro, who did exactly the same. He'd stop me at the door and I had to diagnose the ward by observation. On a good day I might get 27 out of 30, and on a bad day less than 20—but it was great training in observation. After all, Conan Doyle, the creator of Sherlock Holmes, was also a medical student at Edinburgh and modeled the great detective (which, in my opinion, is what a doctor must be) on Sir Joseph Bell, the surgeon of "Bell's palsy" fame.

My specialist exams for the Royal College of Physicians came in three parts, a year apart and finally, if you passed, I think that out of 300 doctors who started, only 30 survived.

I stayed in the Victoria League with other students from all around the world. In the room opposite were two Chinese students. I'd study until 4 a.m. but never was their light off when I turned in. They were encyclopedias of medicine. Such was the competition.

And so I resorted to my native cunning, which Clarrie had reinforced: "Common things occur most commonly." This is a well-known medical axiom and also one of the most ignored. But I needed it so as to compete with my Chinese encyclopedic insomniacs, and it worked. Both the examiners of the Royal Colleges of Medicine in Edinburgh and London, while putting me through a psy-war trial of tricks and false trails, did not find me wanting and I passed.

I do not relate this saga for any purposes of self-aggrandizement, as I am sure the Chinese insomniacs sailed through with consummate ease. Rather I am saying that my approach recognized the more important big picture rather than the encyclopedia of minutiae. When it came to the topic of living longer, this meant concentrating on those illnesses that can actually be prevented or cured. The most "common thing" that will kill us prematurely is cardiovascular disease—heart attacks and strokes—and *this* therefore gets top priority, to my way of thinking. Thereafter I address all preventable illnesses in the order they occur.

Time has not only given me more perspective, it has further confirmed my original information and recommendations. Having worked and studied around the world, I feel I have seen the best on offer; no country has a monopoly on talent or information. Prevention has always been my intense interest, which I have pursued from my earliest days in practice.

I then realized that doctors think they already know it all, or, in truth, are so busy they are increasingly limited to their own specialty and are time-poor. So it dawned on me that it was too important to restrict the information in this book to that of another medical text. Therefore I have rewritten it for the public—by which I mean those people who are motivated to look after themselves and want the best information to do so.

My approach is simple: addressing what's going to kill us prematurely and how can we avoid such causes of death and disability. By identifying these illnesses in prioritized order and by accessing the latest and best medical evidence, this prevention now can be done.

Mileham Hayes, Thornton 2017

THE SEVEN AGES OF MAN

All the world's a stage,
And all the men and women merely players;
They have their exits and their entrances,
And one man in his time plays many parts,
His acts being seven ages. At first, the infant,
Mewling and puking in the nurse's arms.
Then the whining schoolboy, with his satchel
And shining morning face, creeping like snail
Unwillingly to school. And then the lover,
Sighing like furnace, with a woeful ballad
Made to his mistress' eyebrow. Then a soldier,
Full of strange oaths and bearded like the pard,
Jealous in honor, sudden and quick in quarrel,
Seeking the bubble reputation
Even in the cannon's mouth. And then the justice,
In fair round belly with good capon lined,
With eyes severe and beard of formal cut,
Full of wise saws and modern instances;
And so he plays his part. The sixth age shifts
Into the lean and slippered pantaloon,
With spectacles on nose and pouch on side;
His youthful hose, well saved, a world too wide
For his shrunk shank, and his big manly voice,
Turning again toward childish treble, pipes
And whistles in his sound. Last scene of all,
That ends this strange eventful history,
Is second childishness and mere oblivion,
Sans teeth, sans eyes, sans taste, sans everything.

As You Like It, Act II Scene VII. Shakespeare.

It is contended that if we can predict the illnesses and changes, as detailed in The Missing Keys, we may avoid the sixth and seventh stages or minimize and compress them at least.

Live Longest – Book 1: The Missing Keys

Table of Contents

Section 1:

Identifying

The Missing Keys

1. The Long Journey Health Plan

If we set out on a long trip we automatically plan our route and check for any known or potential problems. We would no more go blindly to some war zone, terrorist high-risk hotspot or epidemic area, than fly to the Moon. By contrast, while we do seek attention for an acute illness, most of us don't even have a vague "long journey" health plan other than the practically useless annual check-up. In addition, most of us indulge in high-risk behaviors, which we don't realize or simply ignore. While we know smoking is bad, we don't really think of our overeating, not exercising, sunbaking on holidays or fast driving style as being "high-risk." And our peers and community often condone much high-risk behavior, such as the Friday night binge.

If you want to live longest and best, the 12 fundamental high-risk behaviors must be addressed. Some are insidious, such as quad bikes—great fun but the now the greatest cause of farm deaths. Some are in denial, such as unsafe sex. Deep-sea fishing is found to be the most dangerous occupation; of course, while we all have to earn a living, we can assess the occupational risks involved and, if there are risks, try and find another safer job. Medicine is high-risk, as the high burnout and suicide rates attest, and most clinicians don't seek help. Illicit drugs are simply madness, not just for the deleterious effects of the active ingredient but because of the unknown contaminants. Drugs made by an approved manufacturer have to pass stringent quality and content controls, but the street and party drugs can be made by anyone with no idea of chemistry or hygiene.

More people are killed on the roads than in wars. Young men in overpowered fast cars—let alone when fueled with alcohol—are accidents just waiting to occur. Motorbikes have no protection and, even if you are a safe and careful driver, the truck driver may not be and the bus may not see you. Motorbikes account for 5% of motor vehicles but 25% of accidents. While the motorbike riders are becoming more aggressive, challenging and daring the cars, the cars are bigger and will survive better.

Jogging is good, but for goodness' sake, jog *into* the oncoming traffic on the "wrong" side of the road so you can see what's coming and not be run down from behind. One of my rugby team was the fastest winger I've ever seen and destined for international selection until he was run over from behind while jogging.

Long-Term Lethal

My point here is that many of us become, if not trapped, then acclimatized to the risks of our jobs, hobbies and lifestyles and downplay or even accept them. I am not advocating living in a cocoon, but like a good poker player you should know the risks and percentages. Then you are in the best, informed position to make a decision. It is, of course, up to you to decide to go base jumping, crew on an Alaskan trawler or fly a gyrocopter; but you should be fully informed of the risks. While these pursuits are obviously high-risk, when it comes to eating pizza and being unfit we simply don't place our behavior in the same "high-risk" category. Yet the long-term consequences lead to our premature deaths or up to 20 years as a nursing home invalid. The risks may seem inconsequential at the time but they are long-term lethal.

Do I speak from experience? Well, yes. I have had drug-addicted and suicided colleagues. I knew world-renowned musicians who died from "stepped-on" (adulterated) heroin. I am the only person I know who owned a motorbike and didn't have an accident (but I parked it on the side of the road and sold it then and there after nearly being beheaded). I had a gay relative who died, too young, from emphysema from chain smoking but never got HIV; while his partner did, from a one-night stand. One person I knew simply "disappeared" (overboard) while sailing: they were a *very* hard drinking crew. I don't know any gyrocopter pilots or hang gliders but I have done a fair amount of gliding—with a world-accredited pilot. Did I drive too fast? Well BP (British Petroleum) offered to sponsor me at 19 when I bought my first Porsche (I was a highly paid musician as well as a medical student) and, according to my wife I still drive too fast; but I now let her drive me (so I'm not all that dumb). I've had numerous broken ribs but still ran large teaching hospitals as the only doctor on at night or weekends. I rode a bike for 7 years to school and soon understood to defer to cars.

My father graduated in medicine in 1924, well before antibiotics and when vitamins were being discovered; he advocated (rather than preached) natural foods, saying to me when I was just a little boy: "It is the processing and refining of food that is the problem." And so, while drinking soft drinks and sodas, eating lollipops, candies, ice-cream and cake like any 7-year-old, the main bulk of our food was fresh. I never developed a "sweet tooth" and progressively had less and less of the junk. Just yesterday my wife said how she couldn't remember her last soda / soft drink and neither could I.

It has been found that adult eating habits are the best examples for children. By no means was I a strict Mediterranean Dieter but in the main it was a fresh-food diet even though it was also high in meat. No one can say for certain if this has resulted in my low LDL cholesterol and reasonably good coronary arteries, but it sure didn't harm me. Would I be stricter now that I know even more? You betcha! Now I stick pretty much to the ***Newtrition PHYTO Diet (Book 2)***, eating what are the medically evidenced beneficial foods.

While herd immunity is the modern catchphrase, I was brought up to wash my hands. The Ebola epidemic is a timely reminder. Surgical site infections should be less than 2%, and when I exceeded this I noticed that my assistants did not scrub up for the required time. Since reinforcing this rule I can't remember a wound infection. I was brought up to practice hygiene with respect to food preparation and to be careful as to what I ate—especially when traveling overseas; whereas my best man tried to go native and eat the local, undercooked food, and got amoebic dysentery, then growths on his heart valve, with dire consequences.

These are all common sense and, in the main, well known good Lifestyle practices. However, even if we did practise them, there have also been "Missing Keys" which, despite our best efforts, can come out of left field to unexpectedly and prematurely kill or disable us.

These "Missing Keys" are the illnesses, conditions or accidents that most affect us at certain stages of our lives: They are, to a great degree, "age specific". Suicide, alcohol, drugs, pregnancy mishaps occur in our 20s and early 30s. Then the heart attacks and problems start followed by cancers.

If we could, *and now we can,* identify these most likely fatal or debilitating illnesses for our present age then, at last, we stand the best chance of avoiding or preventing them.

These are now identified for you and presented in separate chapters for men and women arranged in the different age groups.

Then, preventive or avoidance advice, according to the latest and best medical evidence, is provided.

2. The Daily Unrealized High-Risk, Life-Shortening Behaviors:

Risk Factor %	Males % of Total Burden	Females % Total Burden
Tobacco smoking	12.1%	6.8%
Physical Inactivity	6	7.5
High Blood Pressure	5.1	5.8
Alcohol harm	6.6	3.1
Overweight	4.4	4.3
Lack of Fruit / Veg	3.0	2.4
High Cholesterol	3.2	1.9
Illicit Drugs	2.2	1.3
Unsafe Sex	1.1	0.7

HIGH-RISK BEHAVIOR	QUICK FIX
Tobacco–cigarette smoking	Support & nicotine replacement; ?e-cigs
Processed foods, lack fruit / vegetables	Adopt Newtrition PHYTO Foods (Book 2)
Exercise patterns – physical inactivity	Try the 10-20-30 or HIT Plan (Book 4)
High blood pressure	Get checked. Lose weight. No salt or sugar
Drinking habits – alcohol harm	Reduce to 1 to 2 glasses a day
Weight – overweight	Intermittent Fasting Diets (Book 4)
High LDL	Get checked. Adopt Newtrition PHYTO Diet
Driving style	Independent opinion. Don't speed
Hobbies – high risk	Base jumping, Mt Everest – are you serious?
Occupations – high risk	Outdoors, machinery, quad bikes, sports
Unsafe sex	HIV kills, other STDs are on the increase
Illicit drugs	Are you serious? Just don't do it
UVR – ultraviolet – sun damage	Cover up
Not being vaccinated	Author's addition. Vaccinate for everything
Hygiene – poor	Author's addition. See later Book
Environmental pollution	Author's addition. Trees. Shut car windows
Head trauma from sport	Author's addition. Tennis anyone?

Youth High Risk Behavior (US high school students) [3]

The following shows the extent as to just how pervasive and insidious are such high risk behaviors and at such a young age does not bode well for their future.

- 42% reported texting or emailing while driving
- 17% had used prescription drugs (e.g., OxyContin, Xanax) without a prescription at least once.
- Among sexually active teens (30%), just 57% had used condoms during their last sexual intercourse
- 15% had been bullied electronically, 20% had been bullied at school
- 9% had attempted suicide in the past year
- 5% had not eaten fruit
- 7% had not eaten vegetables
- 14% had not been physically active during the past week
- 11% smoked but 25% used electronic cigarettes

While the message that smoking kills has led to falling numbers of smokers in all informed Western countries, the message about the effects of other high-risk behaviors has been less successful. While obesity was only realized as being a developing problem in 1985, nutrition became a hot topic in the 1950s when Ancel Keys pointed out that the Mediterranean peoples had less heart attacks; he ascribed the high rate of heart attacks in Britain and the United States to their diet high in saturated fats. There is now debate as to this conclusion, but there is little doubt that processed foods—high in sugar, salt and additives and low in natural vitamins or minerals—have ushered in the modern Diseases of Affluence—obesity, blood pressure, hyperlipidemia, diabetes 2 and their sequela of cardiovascular disease (heart attacks and strokes), osteoarthritis and depression.

After smoking I would rank processed foods as the second high-risk behavior but globally poor diet, not necessarily processed, comes first

It is important to understand that being overweight or underweight, eating processed and fried foods, and binge drinking are also high-risk behaviors like smoking, drunk driving and speeding. More than 50% of the factors that adversely affect our health are due to behaviors such as cigarette smoking, poor eating, drinking and exercise patterns.

A “toxic environment” no longer means one where there has been a radiation leak or chemical spill. We now live in a “toxic food environment” where all the wrong kinds of food are available 24 hours a day, 7 days a week. Much of this food is "energy dense" but "nutrient deficient"—that is, high in calories but low in nutritional benefits.

In the Sun Belt zones, whites live in an ultraviolet toxic environment. It may seem far-fetched to call something like sunbathing high-risk behavior, but it is. Skin cancer is now an epidemic among white-skinned people in Sun Belt areas, and it is a problem even in Europe. Greater affluence and mobility has resulted in more Europeans holidaying and sun-baking in Spain and other sunny holiday destinations, increasing that risk (except for the case of Swedish women who, with regular sun exposure, paradoxically, live longer).

There are a number of examples, albeit few, which demonstrate the effectiveness of preventive medicine if and when it is put into practice. North Karelia in Finland had the world's highest rate of heart deaths. Through community effort and cooperation, between 1970 and 1997, they dropped their death rate by 75%—faster than anywhere else in Europe. In that time their cholesterol declined by 19%. This is arguably the most successful community demonstration of preventive medicine at work, but it did involve almost total community support and cooperation without, it would seem, the interference of commercial or vested interests.

Ireland also achieved good results in the 15 years between 1985 and 2000, when deaths from coronary heart disease dropped by 47%. A decrease of 40% can be put down to treatments effects and secondary prevention, and 48% to better trends in risk factors—specifically, the prevalence of smoking dropped by 25%, cholesterol concentrations by 30%, and blood pressure by 6%.

These two examples show it can be done.

However, in 2015, the WHO reported that Ireland, by 2030, is predicted to have rates of overweight as high as 89% among men and 85% among women (with three in every four men and two in every three women in the United Kingdom) so it would seem a short honeymoon.

Unfortunately, however, most interventions designed to encourage people to change high-risk behavior have been, to date, either not very successful or overwhelmingly disappointing, despite monumental effort and costs.

The MRFIT study is a good example. The study conducted in 1980 cost US$180 million and was probably the most intensive and expensive clinical trial ever to try and get people to change their behavior. These participants were carefully selected, highly motivated and well informed; but the study could be said to have been an overwhelming failure.[62] These people wanted to stop smoking, reduce their cholesterol, get fit and do what had to be done. They volunteered! They were counseled, coddled, encouraged and monitored, but for some reason most dropped out. Cost was not a factor as the program was free. It was a very disappointing result.

The efforts of the World Health Organization, governments, organized religion, and other authorities have been similarly underwhelming.

This lack of success at the macro level highlights the importance of the individual and the clinician working at the micro level with individual patients on a daily basis. The physician has a prime responsibility, indeed an obligation, to influence his patients and target those at risk.

And so we move through life in our own community with no real forward planning as to our health; and any illness often comes as a complete surprise. Some people feel that by being super-fit and eating what they think are healthy foods, that they are doing all that is necessary...pity about those heart attacks out of the blue. I've heard, many times, "He was so fit," about a 40-year-old who suddenly dies. In fact my old rugby halfback was the surfing ironman and legendary cross-country champion, but one day he just didn't come back from his run.

But Further:

The Missing Keys now identifies the other major conditions, specific to our sex and present age, which are The Missing Keys that lead to our Premature Death or Disability.

What Doesn't Kill You Makes You Stronger

The old adage (I think it was Nietzsche) that "what doesn't kill you makes you stronger" is rubbish! Balderdash! Because most of those conditions that don't kill us leave us disabled.

By identifying these Missing Keys we can then take avoiding or preventive action.

The Causes of Premature Deaths and Disabilities in the USA, England and Wales and Australia but applicable to all first world countries are identified in prioritized, official National Lists. The tables go past 80 years of age, which is the object of Live Longest - Compression of Morbidity - "Living Healthier Longer".

The conditions that cause Death and Disabilities are often the same but can be very different. Cancer is invariably fatal and so the associated disabilities are much the same: whereas Anxiety or Depression, while causing a great deal of Disablement, are not invariably fatal: The sufferer lives much longer and relatively few die.

While Death or Disability before 80 years of age can now be viewed as "Premature", thereafter they are not. At present around 114 years would seem as long as we can live but this is exceptional.

While the search is on for Longevity by a number of different scientific approaches this ignores The Missing Keys - those illnesses which are preventable or avoidable and prematurely kill or disable us. It is not much use having gene therapy, stem cells, young blood, being cryo-vacced or whatever, if you have Cardiovascular Disease, Cancer, Alzheimer's they are not much use to you...and certainly of no use now, whereas The Missing Keys gives you the best chances of Living Longest ***now.***

Summary: To live longest:

1. **Reduce Risks - High-risk Behaviors**:
   - Tobacco – cigarette smoking
   - Processed foods
   - Physical inactivity
   - High blood pressure
   - Drinking habits – alcohol harm
   - Lack of fruit & vegetables
   - Weight – overweight/underweight
   - High LDL (Cholesterol)
   - Driving style
   - Hobbies – high-risk
   - Occupations – high-risk (pesticides, diesel, sun exposure)
   - Unsafe sex
   - Illicit drugs
   - Excessive ultraviolet light (sun) exposure, especially for whites
   - Poor hygiene
   - Lack of vaccinations
   - Head trauma from sport
   - Air pollution
   - Traffic (car) noise

2. **Maximize Health Prevention and Avoidance Protocols**
   - ***Missing Keys:*** Identify illnesses most likely to be encountered
   - Get it seen: Get it diagnosed: Get It Better
   - Tests and Investigations as per Section 4
   - Beneficial Foods: Adopt Newtrition PHYTO Diet
   - Successful Aging Techniques - Socialize - Finances - Lifestyle
   - Exercise
   - Optimize Weight
   - Meticulous attention to and control of any illnesses / conditions

3. What You Are Going to Die From and How to Avoid Them

"Death in old age is inevitable but death before old age is not."
Sir Richard Doll, 1994

Sir Richard Doll was the "foremost epidemiologist of the 20th century" and "perhaps Britain's most eminent doctor" (*BMJ*). His most significant work was on smoking, which he thought caused lung cancer; he quit smoking in 1950. He died aged 92 after a short illness—heart failure.

What's Going to Kill or Cripple You This Week? The Bad News.

Do you know what serious illnesses you are most likely to encounter this month or this year, let alone what specific illness is most likely to strike you right now?

And, if you did know, wouldn't you seek the best information and advice as to how to avoid that illness?

Many people manage to keep fit—whether from jogging, running ultra-marathons or pumping iron—and many make sure to eat the healthiest foods. Many are diligent with annual medical check-ups. However, most people, and in fact, most doctors, simply don't know the lists of what illnesses are most likely at your age. Some, of course, have a good idea; but when I asked my clinical colleagues, whose ages ranged from their 20s to their 80s, they couldn't give an accurate, decade-by-decade list for either women or men. How then can they address the age-specific preventable threats to your health?

Are Annual Medical Check-Ups Helpful?

A 2012 systematic review (14 clinical trials, 182,000 patients followed for av. 9 years) revealed that well patients derived no benefit from an annual physical exam.[4] Yet some 44 million Americans a year take part in this medical ritual of visiting the doctor for an annual physical.[5]

The Good News

The good news is that there are now official specific and detailed lists of what kills or debilitates us at what age, decade by decade, and for both sexes. This data has been diligently and painstakingly gathered by most Western nations' government health departments. It gives us the most information as to how we are likely to die; and, more importantly, it can guide us as to how to avoid such causes of death. No one can know exactly how they will die, but at least you now have the best chance of avoiding a premature death or being an invalid.

The lists are from the United States, United Kingdom, and Australia, with input from most First World countries, and despite minor differences they are applicable to all First World nations. Lists are ordered in priority from the most likely illness as number one, right through to number 20 or more. The most critical data indicates the most likely *Causes of Death*. Then there is the other most important list of most likely *Causes of Disabilities*. Additional lists cover the *Prevalent Health Problems and Why We Visit the Doctor*, then *The Most Commonly Reported Long-Term Conditions*—which, while they don't kill or disable us, reduce our quality of life.

Decade-by-Decade Changes in Illnesses: The Missing Key

Until now this information has been the "Missing Key" for living healthier and longer. Now, however, identifying the illnesses most likely to strike us down, focused at our specific age, allows for the most complete overall picture of our health. It is basic common sense that, if we know just what illnesses are most likely to strike, then we can take the most appropriate, specific investigations and focused, preventive actions to avoid them.

What Else Will Kill Me?

Let's find out and get on the front foot to prevent them, and not just treat illnesses *after* they have occurred.

Specific Tailored Prevention

This unique contribution allows for prevention designed specifically for you, to allow you to address the most important immediate health issues, now, so you can live longer and healthier.

All Ages

This book is for everyone, of all ages, from before 10 to after 100.

Why Hasn't This Been Done Before?

If it is so obvious, why hasn't this "Missing Key" shown up before? This is explained later but, in essence, there are many players eager for your "health dollar," even manipulating and interfering in health, such that the doctor is now well down the list, at number eight in fact. Most people only go to the doctor when they are ill and not for preventive advice. The information in this book has only become available relatively recently; yet it is so obvious as to prompt us to say, "Why didn't I think of that?"

Get With the Evidence: Most Illnesses Can Be Prevented

Most major illnesses can be prevented by nutrition and lifestyle. There have been profound, legitimate, evidenced surveys, trials and studies, which have now been updated in the information here. Most of the recommendations are simple and do not cost any more than what you are doing already. These recommendations are provided in detailed, referenced, evidenced plans and programs after your specific age-related risks are identified.

Not many of us are willing and able to discipline ourselves to a joyless, spartan lifestyle with unproven, unnecessary, expensive vitamins and supplements, buckets of antioxidants (which may be bad for you), or whatever else pseudo-science "health" books and regimes promote. But in any case this is not the advice advocated here.

Instead this book provides simplified, authoritative information, and an approach that is eminently pleasant and achievable—as opposed to having to visit multiple medical specialists; trying an Internet search of dubious, confused or conflicting advice by commercial or vested interests; or reading a book by some unqualified young "wellness guru." There are, of course, some inescapable facts; we can't sit and eat milk chocolate and pizzas all day while watching TV. What can be done is the gradual introduction of changes, making pleasant, acceptable substitutions of good for bad—foods, activities, habits and lifestyles—with the reassurance that the information is the absolute best available.

Disaster can still strike us out of the blue. No one can claim 100% prevention. But even these sudden health crises can be minimized.

Not all illnesses can be prevented; but why not prevent those that can be?

Not Dead, Just Disabled... For 20 Years

If the heart attack, the cancer or the depression doesn't actually kill the person, they then invariably end up as "disability cripples," confined to a long, slow, 10-to-20-year, inexorable, downhill demise. There are premature deaths and then there are premature disabilities. In fact CDC data from the 2014 National Health Interview Survey has found that that a quarter of US adults have at least two chronic conditions. The conditions in question are arthritis, asthma, cancer, chronic obstructive pulmonary disease, coronary heart disease, diabetes, hepatitis, hypertension, stroke, and renal weakness or failure.[6] Most of these can be avoided and certainly better controlled.

Many seriously ill patients consider some debilitating conditions as even worse than death, (*JAMA Internal Medicine* 2016):

1. Bowel and bladder incontinence
2. Relying on a breathing machine to live
3. Being unable to get out of bed
4. Being confused all the time
5. Having to rely on a feeding tube to live
6. Needing care all the time

Quality of Life (QOL)

In addition to longevity, quality of life is examined. Impediments such as deafness and degenerating eyesight are common and not "minor." It is not much fun being otherwise healthy but totally socially isolated or handicapped; so preventing such issues is also addressed.

Live Longest – Complete Health Plan

Live Longest is a series of books that cover all aspects of today's health, from high-powered advanced advice on cardiovascular disease to complementary alternative medicine. This first book covers the essentials, and thereafter many other subjects are covered in much greater detail. These are listed at the end of this book.

This is not just another health or lifestyle book.

It is the product of over 50 years of cumulative hard medical research and clinical experience. It provides you with the "Missing Keys" to predict and thus avoid the illnesses proven most likely for your age.

You now have access to the best percentages, evidence, and systematic plan for how to stay healthy, living well and as long as possible

4. Preventive Maintenance

The Concept of Preventive Maintenance

Scheduled, routine preventive maintenance for airplanes is well understood and accepted. It is totally inconceivable to any of us that we would fly in planes that have not been regularly inspected, tuned, serviced and tested. The wisdom of regular preventive maintenance of our cars is also appreciated. Why is it then that we don't extend the same preventive maintenance principles to our own bodies? It very often takes a health scare before we do anything about looking after ourselves properly. In fact, most of us spend more money on regularly servicing our cars, getting regular haircuts or beauty treatments than we do on our own health.

On the other hand, many spend huge amounts of money on trying to be healthy by buying vitamins, supplements, special diets and gym memberships. These strategies may or may not be necessary or even healthy; in any event, they can possibly be improved given the correct medical evidence rather than a commercial sales pitch.

Waiting until we are ill before we visit the doctor is simply the way it has always been. Understandably, we don't visit the doctor when we are well, only when we are sick.

Why go when we are well? As previously pointed out, a 2012 review revealed that well patients derived no benefit from an annual physical exam—the old routine "annual check-up" which just goes through the same old "one size fits all" examination and tests.

However, like any machine, different parts of humans wear out at different times; different illnesses affect us at different ages. This new information now allows us to match a patient's age with their age-specific illnesses. And while we may wait until we are sick to visit the doctor, this is rather like waiting for your car to break down before you get it seen to. There is a better way to look after our bodies and optimize our health—Preventive Medical Maintenance—in the same way we look after our cars and planes.

What I advocate, rather than a one-size-fits-all annual physical, are regular check-ups specific to your age and sex, as per the documented death and disability tables.

The evidence from the advances in medical research is that regular but *focused, specific medical checks* can nip problems in the bud. These medical checks *concentrate on what conditions are most likely to affect you for your age and sex.* This approach gives you the best chance of "curing most known diseases," optimizing our health and increasing our lifespan by up to 15 or more years.

Analysis of the new evidence as to what health problems affect us for each decade of our lives has allowed *the development of age-specific health recommendations and a health "preventive maintenance service schedule."* The intent is not only to look for illnesses but also to identify risks that can be minimized to help *prevent* them. Based on your age and sex, specific focused risks can be identified and warnings flagged to institute appropriate avoidance/preventive measures, as well as overall health. What needs to be done to service our cars and flag warnings is different at 5,000 km, 20,000 km or 100,000 km; and so the required medical service differs for us at the ages of 30, 40, 50 years and beyond.

This approach then allows selection of *the most appropriate preventive measures, tests and investigations specific to your age.* You can continue like most people to see a doctor only if you have a problem—but that works only after you have done your Preventive Maintenance. The human body does not remain as we were at 11 years of age. Ignorance is not medical bliss.

The illnesses or causes of death for a 20-year-old male are different from those of a man aged 60. Women have a different set of age-specific illnesses, sometimes nearly the same as for men but sometimes widely different, as the tables show. Of course any acute illness should be seen to immediately and completely fixed, as discussed later.

In addition to age-specific preventive measures *there are also universal recommendations for optimizing our health* and therefore our longevity, which apply to all of us at any time in the lifespan. These involve the correct nutrition or diet, the correct exercise and lifestyle. Above all these should be pleasant and acceptable, not a rigorous, spartan imposition.

Below are two pictures of the same model, same year, 1928 Rolls Royces.

Before moving past the analogy of regular car servicing, allow me to illustrate the basic principles of preventive health maintenance. The car in the first picture has been regularly serviced and maintained; the other hasn't. Which one is most like you?

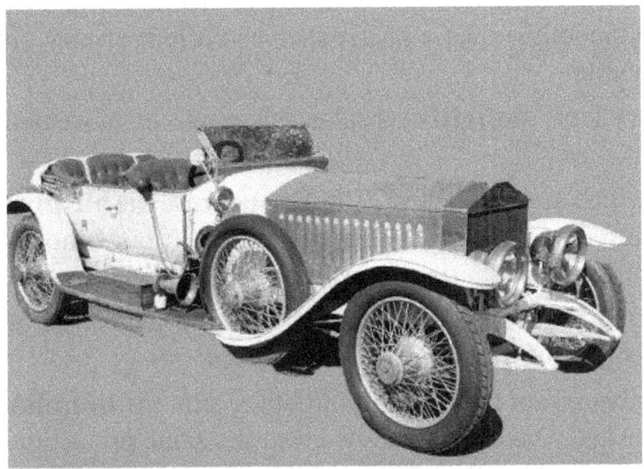

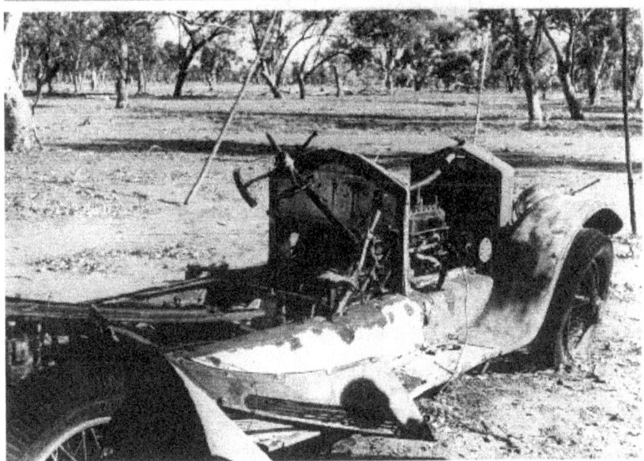

The successfully aged Rolls had the **best fuel and oil** put into it, which equates to the best **nutrition or foods** for a human. The world's best-evidenced foods, which I have called "New"trition, are detailed later. Again this solution is pleasant and acceptable to all.

An **engine** which has been regularly tuned and not stressed is the equivalent of us having our **heart** checked.

Clean **headlights** with new bulbs, the equivalent of looking after our **eyes.**

Correct loading, so the **suspension** has not been stressed, is the equivalent of us keeping our **weight** down, and not pushing beyond limits, so that we do not overly strain our spine and joints.

An **electrical system** and steering that has been immaculately maintained is the equivalent of our **nervous system** being kept tuned and not poisoned with toxins such as alcohol. New spark plugs make the engine run smoothly—like a pacemaker or radiofrequency ablation for our aging hearts.

No **rust**... no **arthritis**: regular full range of movements, gentle mobilization.

Tires, which are in splendid condition because the **air pressure** has been monitored and kept at the optimum level. If our **blood pressure** is checked on a regular basis, our arteries will also be in good condition.

Regular maintenance of the **air filter** and avoidance of airborne pollutants equates to similar care of our **lungs**.

Having been kept garaged and out of the sun, the **upholstery** is not faded or cracked. Our **skin** is rarely given the same protection and most of us have sun- and weather-damaged skin.

A working **horn**, because it has not been overused. Our **voice** and **ears** will benefit from the same treatment.

Having been immaculately kept **clean**—whereas we are inclined to take a casual approach to personal **hygiene**. Rashes, fungal infections, cracked heels, skin lesions abound.

Preventive maintenance and the early identification and repair of even trivial problems has resulted in this car remaining in great condition throughout its life due to Preventive Maintenance, the principles of which can be transferred to our own care.

Continuing the analogy, the beautifully maintained car has only ever been serviced by qualified Rolls Royce mechanics, familiar with the model, who have only used genuine spare parts when repairing the car, and have never used additives or made modifications that haven't been proven to work for the car. Yet, by contrast, we gobble down vitamins and supplements which we should not need and may even damage us; or we try alternative therapies of unproven worth by unqualified "gurus" – the equivalent to unproven fuel additives and backyard mechanics. Few of us would treat our cars like that.

Human Applications

Finally, in cars different systems are checked for each 5000 km or similar thresholds. Not every system is checked each time, and this analogy applies to humans. Since new evidence provides specific information for each decade and sex, a set of specific risks, and appropriate tests and investigations, can be recommended in place of the generic annual or corporate check-up. Regular age-specific Preventive Medical Maintenance optimizes and maximizes health, successful aging and longevity.

5. Why This Book Had to Be Written

The Young Widows of Coronary Care

Appointed as the Intern-Resident Medical Officer for the world's first Coronary Care Unit,7 I became consummately frustrated at being summonsed every night at two, three and four a.m. for what, I came to realize, were often eminently preventable heart attacks. At those god-forsaken, lonely hours, in cold hospital corridors, I often then had to issue the ghastly news, most often to distraught, tragically young widows and their kids, of their husbands' and fathers' sudden and unexpected deaths. There is no "grief counseling" for doctors, so I found it quite distressing—more so because most of these deaths could have been prevented. I did not feel sorry for myself (well, occasionally I did) but I sure as hell felt anguish every time for these families now suddenly deprived of their husband and father.

Fifty years later, despite being more preventable, heart disease is still one of our greatest causes of death. "Analysis of (the last) two decades reveals risk factors are on the rise, despite greater awareness... Despite increased understanding of heart disease risk factors and the need for preventive lifestyle changes, patients are suffering the most severe type of heart attack at a younger age, and they are more likely to have preventable risk factors."[1] Everywhere I still see "heart attacks looking for somewhere to happen" and others who, while they look fit and healthy, still have heart attacks. In the same newspaper urging us to work "past 90" the death was announced of the ex-brother-in-law of one of the world's greatest actresses. He was a handsome, fit-looking American businessman, aged only 46, who "suddenly and very unexpectedly died of a heart attack while in New York," leaving behind his former wife and four children. Yet, 50 years later—after men have gone to the Moon; after color TV, heart transplants, the Internet and iPhones; after the actual treatment for heart attacks has improved—we still have these "sudden and unexpected" heart attacks and deaths.

But most of them now can and *should be* prevented.

---

[1] Report to the American College of Cardiology's 65th Annual Scientific Session, 2016.

50 Years Banging My Head Against a Brick Wall

As I write this, most of my friends and colleagues are around 75 years old and, despite the fact that they include medical professors, world-renowned surgeons, world-champion sportsmen and the nation's foremost vitamin and homeopathic guru, they are dropping like flies. Those left alive are spiraling downwards toward being shambling, senile, multiple medication-taking invalids. They are then confined to nursing homes with "tubes in every orifice" for the next 10 to 20 years, if they are "lucky."

While 75 may be the age some select to die, is this what you want? Or, is this what you want to avoid?

By the very nature of their considerable achievements, those friends of mine were an arrogant lot. Most doctors think they know more than their colleagues. Champion sportspeople have strange diets and stranger rituals, if not superstitions. So both of these groups certainly never sought my advice. I also had other friends who embraced supplements, mostly unproven (and many disproven), while vehemently ignoring evidenced medical advice. This is crazy. It is like believing putting "special" expensive water rather than gasoline in your car will not only work but also work better. One swore by Saw Palmetto, an extract from the Florida Palm, which was meant to prevent prostrate trouble. It does not. Another swore by paw-paw (papaya) oil or juice, because of its enzyme, papain, which tenderizes meat. Another ate yeast and lecithin... and on and on. These are silly beliefs which people adopt, seduced by commercial scams such as the vitamin industry. Yet evidence shows that taking too much beta-carotene, vitamin A or vitamin E may increase mortality,[8] and excess folic acid or vitamin B_{12} may contribute to autism. Even the latest research into vitamin C found that natural sources (fruit and vegetables) were more beneficial than tablets (most of which are made in industrial factories from coal tar—but hey, who do you believe?).

None of these friends listened to me. Patients, let alone friends, don't see the doctor for preventive advice (with the exception that I did get them all to give up smoking). All of them have died prematurely or now have debilitating confining illnesses. Sure, most avoided their heart attacks by not smoking and being fit; but they thought this was enough (plus their supplements). There are, however, many less dramatic evidenced lifestyle changes that accumulate to offer greater protection across the whole spectrum of illnesses.

The Homeopath-Vitamin Guru had all his amalgams removed and had his photo looking dazzlingly healthy on the Vitamin Companies Brochure, but he thought his vitamins would prevent his heart attack. They did not. He had a heart attack, a dissecting aneurysm, and apparently was a paraplegic for the last 3 years of his life. I'm afraid I was not very subtle when his son rang me with the news, as I facetiously mulled, "I guess he just didn't take enough vitamins."

The National Rugby Captain fancied himself as a modern-day Ernest Hemmingway and indulged in high-risk behaviors. His wonderful physical fitness and coordination preserved him from most physical risks—but he ate "wild" food on his expeditions. He got amoebic dysentery after eating raw crocodile in Zambia, and a rare form of fish poisoning which affected a major heart valve. He then suffered a well-known complication of heart surgery, cerebral emboli, resulting in a minor series of strokes. I would have recommended a more specialized hospital and unit, but he didn't ask me.

Mr. Saw Palmetto has cancer of his bladder, which he says is now cured by his new batch of herbs, which I doubt. Meanwhile the professor of surgery has Parkinson's disease, and the Wimbledon champion sports two artificial hips.

Could I have prevented most or some of these calamities if my friends had listened to me? I'd like to think so. The evidence is there. But having to stand by and witness their decline and fall is both terrible and frustrating. So I determined to get the best information out and as widely distributed as possible.

"You can lead a horse to water, but if you can't get it to float on its back and squirt water in the air you ain't got nuthin'"—to make the old proverb more accurate. Most people are not interested in researching the hard medical evidence and are therefore easy prey for the TV vitamin, weight loss and "health" equipment advertisements. Sir William Osler observed that humans distinguish themselves from animals by their desire to take pills; but this is not the best way for the minimization and

prevention of illnesses. A gym is not necessary, but moderate-to-fast walking is. I hand out information to all my patients about nutrition, which should prevent the majority of heart disease and reduce cancer of the colon, as much as anything known can; but I see the look of disinterest in some of the 20- and 30-year-olds, and I doubt if they even read it on their way to the juice shop, tattoo parlor, gym and latest fad. However, most patients did want more information.

If these were not enough reasons to write and disseminate this book, an eminent American doctor, who advised the president, stated in 2014 that he "hoped to die at 75." I found this death wish depressing, for him, and inaccurate for most of us. What is obviously needed is an alternate opinion based on modern evidence and my longer experience.

My father graduated in medicine before antibiotics and most modern medical advances such as x-rays, MRIs, and organ transplants, though he lived long enough to see and use these. He was a very shrewd clinician who, prior to the advances in medicine we now take for granted, had to use a holistic (a Western medicine word) approach. He incorporated the medicine of psychology, physical methods, and nursing, and he taught me about nutrition. He later became one of the first doctors in the world to use penicillin. He gave up smoking in 1947, as he thought "it caused lung cancer," 3 years before Sir Robert Dole started the world's no-smoking campaign. This and his many other observations–including "sugar and processed food are not good for us"—were some 50 years in advance of what has now been proven. I absorbed his teachings, which were not taught in medical school but do need to be passed on.

At the same time, modern medicine has rocketed ahead with quite incredible advances, such that we can and should live longer and healthier, past 75. Sadly, as we become more "civilized," so the Diseases of Affluence–obesity, cardiovascular disease (heart attacks / strokes / blood pressure), diabetes 2, high cholesterol, depression, arthritis, and I would add, sedentary behavior–have become epidemic. Most of the Western world, including 60% of Americans, are now overweight. Eighty thousand new untested chemicals have been introduced since WW2, many of them into our foods or food chain. The fast-food industry has a budget far greater than any government health scheme, surpassing even the GNP of most countries, while delivering us processed foods with additives 24 hours a day, seven days a week.

Against this onslaught, the only defense we have is accessing the correct information from the world's best studies and adopting their recommendations, which should be both acceptable and pleasant (or people won't incorporate them). Then, if things still go wrong, we should know what are the most appropriate medical procedures and hospitals and where to find them.

Finally, most previous advice has ignored or not incorporated the data as to what illnesses you are most likely to encounter for your present age. How then are you meant to avoid them? This is the Missing Key: a complete Preventive Medicine program and plan for those who actually want to look after themselves in the best ways possible. It is for those self-motivated and interested in being healthy, and living longer and better. There is an analysis of patients later in this book, which shows which "Type of Patient" achieves the best health outcome.

6. Older Better? Younger Smarter? Bottom of the Cliff "Salvage" Medicine

When the older generation of medical practitioners such as Sir Richard and my father studied medicine, it was before antibiotics and "modern medicine" and hence mainly based on nutrition, hygiene and healthy behaviors. And while they later saw the advances of modern medicine, they were also able to observe the downsides of some of the new trends that my generation grew up with.

Junk food is one outstanding example. In their day there was no fast-food—drive-thrus, take-aways, instant meals, home-delivered pizzas, super-sized sodas—which we take as normal. So they could compare the "before and after" effects. This more complete overview allowed them a wider choice of optimal health practices. They knew fruit and vegetables supplied essential vitamins, fiber and micronutrients, and the doctors of that era strongly recommended such a diet. But as Western civilization has progressively offered more processed and junk foods, our ingestion of these essential nutrients has been replaced. The newer factory foods are high in calories but low in essential nutrients, and we now have an epidemic of obesity and the "Diseases of Affluence"—Hyperlipidemia, Hypertension, Heart disease, Diabetes, Arthritis and Depression. Meanwhile our eating of fiber has dropped by 55%, as cancer of the colon increases.

In the previous era meat preserving was usually done just with salt, whereas today the shops are full to overflowing with delicious sausages and preserved meats that are full of chemical preservatives, some of which are suspicious for causing colon cancer. We think of sausages, bacon, and ham as "traditional" good foods... but maybe their modern processing is not. Since WW2 chemicals can be introduced with few restrictions. These additives are only withdrawn after severe or fatal side effects are proven. Meanwhile there are some 80,000 chemicals in "approved" daily use—except no one has approved them.

I hasten to say that this is not a trip into the "good old days," as modern medicine has so much more to offer. In fact one of the most common additives was introduced to prevent food poisoning. Each year 48 million Americans—that's one in every six—becomes sick from contaminated food, of whom 128,000 are hospitalized and 3000 die.[9] Some cases of irritable bowel syndrome can now be traced back to episodes of food poisoning,[10] so the benefits of this additive far outweigh any suspected side effects.

However, I do think it is time to pause and make sure we have not thrown the baby out with the bath water; to rediscover old wisdoms while selecting the best modern medicine has to offer. The older generation of doctors saw how unprocessed food actually saved peoples' lives. Consider the story of rice, where the outer brown layer of rice was taken off ("polished") because white rice appealed more to the consumer. This outer layer contained an essential vitamin, and so people eating white rice suffered an essential vitamin deficiency resulting in heart and nerve disease (beriberi and peripheral neuropathy). This condition was only deduced when chickens suffered these same illnesses when fed white rice left over from a Dutch military hospital in Java, but recovered when fed natural, unprocessed brown rice (after some military martinet banned "civilian" chickens from eating the military white rice). The missing, and then mysterious, compound was called a "vital amine," which came to be shortened to *vitamin*. Later it was discovered that the outer layer of rice was rich in this vitamin B1 known as thiamine. Other vitamin deficiencies were due to impoverished diets, such as in the slums of Glasgow, where cod liver oil, rich in vitamin D, "miraculously" prevented rickets in the children whose families couldn't afford good food and who never saw much sun. My father was brought up in this era and saw these actual miracles of vitamins come to light.

Today such poor diets with vitamin deficiencies are only found in those who cannot afford good food, in an institution where the food preparation destroys the vitamins, or among some food faddists. These are the only people who would now need vitamin supplements.

My father's generation also knew the importance of personal hygiene. Ebola has somewhat woken us up to the importance of personal hygiene and washing our hands; and bird flu and MERS (Middle Eastern Respiratory Syndrome) have alerted us to the dangers of coughing and airborne infections. With the advent of antibiotics we have become blasé and careless about these fundamental prevention techniques, as well as more advanced and sophisticated ones.

My father saw all this and what older medicine had to offer but never sat me down and lectured me. Rather it was bits and pieces dropped here and there to alert me. Now what's old is new again, and it amuses me to watch medical documentaries where my father's recommendations have been "rediscovered" as cutting-edge modern medicine.

"Holistic" is not an Alternative Medicine word but a legitimate Western medicine word defined as "characterized by the treatment of the whole person, taking into account mental and social factors, rather than just the symptoms of a disease." To me even this definition does not go far enough. While the whole person is being considered, he or she is still being treated for an illness. Whereas my philosophy, backed by 50 years of clinical experience, would prefer to keep you healthy by preventing illnesses.

That is not to say all illnesses can be prevented; but a hell of a lot, in fact most, can! You have to know not only what prevents illnesses overall, but also what specific illnesses are most likely to occur, and for what age and sex. Then our targeted focus offers us the best chance to avoid or minimize them.

Somewhere around the 1970s, hospitals started to keep better records as to causes of death. I remember my then superintendent hounding me to fill out these new bureaucratic imposts. As a know-it-all (and insanely overworked) smart-ass, I pointed out to him that "death is never a medical emergency" and objected, as I was so busy with the living, why should I attend to this boring trivia for the government bureaucrats? But the super was such a nice guy that I gave in, became a good boy, and filled out the forms.

I found out, decades later, that it was not such a waste of time. While researching something else, I happened upon the resultant governments reports, and here before me was my epiphany, my Eureka Moment; here was the State of the Nation's Health in all its bureaucratic detail! It was an amazing, marvelous revelation, to me at least.

By the 1990s, better non-hospital death certificates not only recorded what killed us, such as a heart attack, but like the hospitals, also noted other contributing, intercurrent illnesses. For example, if someone was struck by a truck and killed while crossing the road, it was previously just recorded as a motor vehicle accident (MVA) and perhaps a "fractured skull." Now consider that this was a 60-year-old woman who was obese—which helped exacerbate her arthritis and cause her diabetes 2, and led to a heart attack and atrial fibrillation, which may have contributed to her Alzheimer's. She wandered off from her nursing home but, as she was disorientated, she didn't look when crossing the road. Slowed by her arthritis and burden of weight, she was hit by the truck. So her real causes of her death were indeed the MVA and fractured skull / brain damage; but contributing factors included her 1) Obesity, 2) Diabetes, 3) Myocardial infarction, 4) Atrial Fibrillation, and 5) Alzheimer's. It would also be noted she was suffering from 6) Osteoarthritis and 7) Reduced mobility. The fact that she was on multiple drugs, including an anticoagulant which made the bleeding from her brain uncontrollable, would probably not be recorded. Still, these more complete details now allowed identification of seven serious associated illnesses or conditions to provide, at last, what old people actually had wrong with them when they die.

I was alerted to this issue at my first hospital, where I was warned, "Never ask the chief pathologist what was the cause of your patient's death, as he will go ballistic." The pathologist was only too well aware that seriously ill patients had multiple pathologies, all of which contributed to their demise.

I can't say whether any of my personally recorded statistics made it to the final government reports. But they provided, for the first time, a complete picture of what kills us all and contributes to our deaths. I call it an epiphany because I realized, almost in a blinding flash, that these statistics could provide a better, more exquisite, system of health care via focused, individual preventive medicine. At last here was the potential to get ahead of the curve by predicting these illnesses and, in most cases, then prevent or minimize them by modern medicine's advances.

I went on to find that most Western countries had similar statistics, and they were almost the same. Heart disease, for instance, is among the greatest killers in the United States, United Kingdom, Europe, Australia, and New Zealand. The data sets were close enough, in fact, that a Universal Preventive Plan could be recommended.

The statistics showed me that tooth decay is the most prevalent disease; hearing loss is second, and back pain is third. Did you know that? I sure didn't, nor did any of my colleagues. Long- and near-sightedness were the most common long-term reported conditions. While most people visited their doctor for coughs and colds, they were mostly actually treated for high blood pressure, URTIs, vaccinations, depression, lipid disorders, then diabetes. Among the most startling revelations were the graphs of cardiovascular (heart/stroke) disease, blood pressure, cholesterol, diabetes, cancer, lung disease, arthritis and osteoporosis, weight and deteriorating eyesight. All these graphs (which I present in later chapters) rose slowly and gradually from birth but then, at age 40, took off and climbed like a rocket!

It immediately struck me that we should be testing for these conditions at 40, or before, and diagnosing them early to ensure better long-term health. It also occurred to me that we must be doing something wrong for all these diseases to suddenly take off at 40. Maybe earlier prevention habits could delay these onsets or deteriorations. For the first time I knew the exact order as to what illnesses were killing and prematurely disabling us, with a breakdown for each sex and each decade. Did you know suicide is the greatest killer and disabler of young men? Do you know what kills most women of 40 or disables most at 50?

If you and your doctor knew what was most likely to kill or disable you at your present age, wouldn't that alert both of you to investigate and take preventive actions? These are now all listed so you can!

I certainly didn't know what specifically affected each patient for each decade, and neither do most doctors. The tsunami of acute illnesses, the full waiting room, the emergencies, the increasing red tape and new advances all deny clinicians the luxury of this overview. Who could sit back, analyze, and digest all the new information, let alone draw conclusions, let alone develop a system or method to optimize health based on this new information?

By happy chance, I was able to do just that.

It was serendipity. I had my own "health scare" and, unlike my colleagues, had the time to sit and consider it all. I take no kudos or credit for this information. What I have done is identify, cull, edit and assemble the world's best medical evidence and advice into a logical, evidenced age- and sex-specific prevention system.

I have not escaped scot-free. Very few, if any, sail through life without some significant if not serious illness, and mine was a stroke. My illness was the type that was totally unpredictable and unpreventable. I was fit, within all normal medical parameters, and on no medications. I had the good fortune of being trained in the best hospitals, so knew I had to search for and find the best radiologist and neurosurgeon. As a result of their superb training, they did not barge in and operate but elegantly diagnosed that my condition was benign (a vein, not an artery bleed) and determined that I didn't need an operation. I recovered completely without intervention. Well, by "no intervention" I mean I avoided having my skull and brain opened. I did, however, while fully conscious, have a catheter passed from my groin, through my heart, into a thread-wide cerebral (brain) artery, back down, across the other side of my heart and up again via my carotid artery, into the Thalamo-striate Artery on the other side of my brain.

Finding the best doctors and facilities, as I had been trained, is part and parcel of surviving and recovering. There is a huge difference between hospitals and treatments. The basic rule is that a university "teaching" hospital has the best standards, and then the further you go out into the country, the less the expertise and specialized facilities and the greater the morbidity and mortality. Prevention then includes finding out the best hospitals and doctors in your area.

My stroke—a rare kind shared by Sharon Stone, who is younger, and Paul Hogan, who is older than I (both of whom also recovered to keep working)—nevertheless caused my temporary retirement and allowed me the time to research all this. I took a whole month off. That was 25 years ago and allowed me see "the other side," to gain further insight and, I feel, be much better placed to recommend and advise. I certainly learned a lesson, regarding my condition and treatment. Despite all the best advice, information and efforts, disaster can still come out of left field, as happened to me. Had I stayed at the first hospital I was sent to, I would have undergone an unnecessary operation, as they did not have the sophisticated equipment or trained radiologists to accurately diagnose me. Instead my wife rang a colleague and found "the best neurosurgeon," straight back from the Mayo Clinic, and I survived without the surgery.

As to prevention, I don't claim any miracle elixir or special secrets; but I do claim to alert you to those illnesses you are most likely to get at your age, and this gives you, by far and away, the best chances of avoiding them and taking specific preventive measures.

Until recently most screening tests and preventive methods were not proven; so it was, if not unethical, then essentially useless to do them (the annual physical check-up has now been "officially" recognized as such). This new evidence and information, however, at last allowed for early focused-specific diagnosis and Predictive Analysis, along with overall prevention.

Being intensely interested in preventive medicine, I have done my lipids test nearly every year since 1968 after running the Coronary Care Unit and reading the Framingham Report. Due to my father's advice against processed foods, my lipids have been normal for the past 48 years of testing. Now I am certainly not boasting here, as "nemesis follows hubris"; and this does not guarantee me absolution from a heart attack or, obviously, my stroke, but it certainly excuses me from having to take statins or what-have-you.

Some years ago I jotted down "Hayes' Laws of Medicine"—about how to be a good doctor. There was no superior knowledge or arrogance in this. I just tabulated what patients have to go through and what many doctors are not aware of, as they haven't gone through it...

A major operation where not much is explained, being in hospital where the nurses are often too busy, essentials are just out of reach or the tea-lady wakes you just as you get to sleep, having a baby, having a heart attack, being told you have cancer or some terminal illness, suffering the death of your partner or loved one, broken ribs, a long-leg plaster in summer, sitting in Casualty-Emergency and being ignored, the incredible unnecessary noise of hospitals, and so on. These are indignities patients have to suffer, and unless we have experienced or observed them ourselves, we can't know how distressing they can be.

In running the Coronary Care Unit, my Registrar and I noted how, when patients woke from their comas, they were totally disoriented and alarmed. The clock might read 12 o'clock—but in this closed unit, was that 12 a.m. or p.m., and where were they? We arranged for 24-hour clocks, and I tried to get patients to windows as soon as possible, where the sun and sound of birds had a marvelous beneficial effect on their morale and their recovery.

Having experienced much of the above does give me insight to what patients go through. While excellent doctors may pass on excellent advice, only those who have visited "the other side" can truly offer the best firsthand advice. My long and varied experience also has provided me with the overall balance of covering most of life's foibles, problems and illnesses. I assure you I do not possess the longevity gene, nor have I led a low-risk lifestyle (quite the reverse in fact). But underlying it all was a protective diet, and an awareness of what illnesses were likely and how to avoid or prevent them, along with the desire to investigate and find the very best medical treatment when things go awry.

This approach forms the fundamental platform of this book: "Smarter Younger," as in the modern advances in medicine; combined with "Older Wiser," with the objectivity of experience. By no means am I claiming that I am smarter; but the statistical information and the medical improvements and advances certainly help, and by combining the two I feel we have a win-win scenario.

Nor, by any means, am I claiming I stick rigidly to the best possible advice if and when it sets too difficult a standard. Most targets can be modified to acceptable levels with nearly as beneficial results. The Mediterranean Diet, which forms the basis for good eating, is pleasant and easy to adopt. Knowing which exercises are best also helps, but since some are an effort, more gentle substitutes are detailed. What lifestyles optimize aging is easy to determine; and what illnesses are most likely for your age should make you keep a weather eye out.

The incredible impost of "information overload" is causing concern that room for this new information has to be made by pushing out earlier stuff. What is worse is that there are now a plethora, if not an epidemic, of predatory publications, hiding behind legitimate sounding names and flatteringly inviting academics to publish. These academics, who are often judged by the number of publications in their CV, are duped into supplying an article, and worse is to follow. These articles are not properly scrutinized (peer reviewed), and when nonsense articles are submitted they are speedily published, complete with spelling errors. One scientist fed up with this practice wrote a spoof which claimed the discovery of weight-losing ingredients in chocolate. This faux revelation, of course, was taken up by the media and presented as a scientific breakthrough on a talkfest breakfast show.

Other health books I've checked are about keeping fit or offering general health advice. While some are good, these fitness/diet titles ignore the fact that all of us are prone to and usually get certain illnesses at certain ages. Theirs is almost a philosophy of denial, as if heart attacks and cancers don't exist in their super-fit, superfood supplement world. On the other hand, others are "illness" books which concentrate of one illness and advocate strange alternative "cures." They tell you how to recover and beat your diabetes, heart attack, cancer or whatever, but invariably offer false hopes, based on unproven recommendations, to a frightened and terribly vulnerable group.

The recommendations in this book come from the world's best trials and studies. They are peer reviewed and from the world's top 10 or so recognized medical journals.

Some information is given here which has not been conclusively proven, but appears to have some basis in research; for example, cocoa and walnuts having a potential beneficial effect on the lining of our arteries. You are urged to be skeptical but keep an open mind about such suggestions.

Many "health" books, of course, are not written by medical practitioners, let alone clinicians who actually treat ill patients. At best these keep-fit or health books are only half the story. Preventing or minimizing illnesses is the other half. This is eminently possible and what this book is all about. To that end this book presents a unique, definitive approach to long-lasting health for everyone who wishes to grow old and to be as healthy as possible. It is never too late—as we grow older we are prone to inevitable disorders of age but many of these can also be avoided or minimized. It is also never too early—if you are pregnant even your unborn child will benefit from this advice, as in the fruit section in the Newtrition Notes.

Initially, I presented these "revelations" in a series of seminars for the public in 2007 at my old university, which, like most medical schools, doesn't have a Faculty of Preventive Medicine. However, I got waylaid: I was commissioned by the world's largest medical publisher to write a textbook, which then became two major textbooks (on skin cancer and surgery) of some 1,000 pages, which took seven concentrated, grueling years. In this time I thought someone else would surely write this book, as the information was, and is, available to every medical practitioner.

But no one wrote it, or anything like it, which I found most surprising; as this new information made living longer and healthier possible and there was an obvious need. So I sat back and looked at my colleagues—from cardiologists, to other physicians, surgeons, Primary Care and General Practitioners—to see if I could divine a reason for this. Frankly, I was taken aback at their workloads. Some had actually offered to help with my skin cancer and surgery books but there was always some reason why they were too busy when I said that chapter was ready. And they were! They were and are all too busy! I sincerely doubt if any of them have ever looked at the complete National Health Statistics or even know they exist in a digestible form except for their own specialty. Today most doctors are only interested or have time for their particular interest or specialty, and certainly not the overall national decade-by-decade health statistics for both sexes that I happened upon and pored over.

I have a colleague who only operates on hands. If you want your chopped-off fingers sewn back on, he's among the world's best—but don't ask him about anything else. Cardiologists may give good preventive advice, but only for your heart, and not how to prevent cancer of your colon. GPs or Primary Care doctors are simply too busy and need this information served up to them, which, hopefully, I have now done. This book was initially intended for doctors but I realized that by informing the end-user, you the patient, it would have a much wider distribution and use.

Prevention has not progressed because people only go to doctors when they are sick—which had accurately been identified as "Bottom of the Cliff Medicine" more than 120 years ago in a poem by Joseph Malins. Now, at last, we can not only put up a fence but construct a Super-Highway of Health which avoids the cliffs.

The Ambulance Down In The Valley[11]

by Joseph Malins, 1895

'Twas a dangerous cliff, as they freely confessed,
Though to walk near its crest was so pleasant;
But over its terrible edge there had slipped
A duke, and full many a peasant;
So the people said something would have to be done,
But their projects did not at all tally.
Some said: "Put a fence around the edge of the cliff";
Some, "An ambulance down in the valley."

[Final verse of seven:]

Better guide well the young than reclaim them when old,
For the voice of true wisdom is calling;
To rescue the fallen is good, but 'tis best
To prevent other people from falling;
Better close up the source of temptation and crime
Than deliver from dungeon or galley;
Better put a strong fence 'round the top of the cliff,
Than an ambulance down in the valley.

And while it is pure Victorian melodrama, Malins was ahead of his time in advocating "Prevention rather than Picking Up the Pieces." In fact, 121 years ahead of his time, as prevention has never realized its promise or potential, until now. Doctors were and are not sought for prevention, and so preventive medicine became a backwater. As a consequence, not many doctors specialize in prevention, especially at a clinical level; and so there has been no apparent interest in an overview to "put it all together." Rather than Bottom of the Cliff Medicine, I see this *Live Longest* system as analogous to putting up a roadblock and warning lights to stop you from plummeting over the cliff; and what is more, constructing a new alternate route. Stay on the new Super-

Highway To Health and don't plummet over the cliff where, at best, all we can do is pick up and patch. Don't get ill; prevent it by predicting what is most likely and taking evidenced steps to avoid it.

Medicine has become progressively diverse and specialized. There are two main groups: one is the clinicians who actually see, diagnose and treat patients; the other is the non-clinicians, who range from those who actively support clinicians (such as radiologists and pathologists, who occasionally see patients) to those who have abandoned any contact with patients to become researchers such as epidemiologists. This division has led, in my observation and experience, to an unbalanced dichotomy. The clinician is weighed down by the urgent and inescapable demands of patients and is time-poor, while the non-clinician has to "publish or perish"—get articles into journals—to get funding or a better job. The clinician has no time to read this tsunami of often dubious articles (as noted above) while the non-clinician and their camp followers of non-medical graduates are busy creating this tsunami. The result is that many, if not most, clinicians don't access the rare gems hidden in this tsunami—as nearly happened to me. So the clinicians continue seeing patients, and while they keep up with clinical advances they don't read much epidemiology or statistics, let alone prevention articles.

To confirm my observations, as noted before, I asked some colleagues what illnesses they were personally most likely to suffer or die from. My colleagues ranged in age through all decades from 20 to 80, both sexes and most specialties and primary care fields... and none of them knew (except some over 50 who did correctly pick heart disease, and thereafter didn't know). I can't see my colleagues finding the time to source and read all this data, and the medical schools don't teach it, so I have redirected my efforts to you, the motivated individual. While "Prevention" has been my passion, it does not rate a mention when I am asked to confirm my specialty for international surveys whose lists go from "A": Aviation Medicine, to "V": Vascular Surgery, but offer no Prevention in the "P" section. So it would seem that clinicians with an interest in Prevention are thin on the ground. However, as a Specialist Physician, I have researched, thought, mulled over and studied being healthy and preventing illnesses for 50 years, and even longer if I count listening to the observations of my father. And while I went on to work in some of the most advanced, high-powered medical units in the world, these overall, holistic observations were not lost to me. I have been able to scan across the widest field of medicine and provide an evidenced health plan that maximizes our chances of living longer and healthier—past 75.

Where ***Live Longest*** differs from any other book is that it not only address the optimum lifestyles for longevity, it also recognizes that everyone gets ill and so identifies the illnesses most likely to occur at your age, and how to avoid or minimize them. Included is the priority of those conditions most likely to affect you, which alters for each sex and from decade to decade. This is a unique Total Health Package of benefit to all.

7. How Computers and the Government Can Help You (Inadvertently) with Big Data: Analyze, Predict, Prevent

The development of computers has enabled the crunching of "big data," which allows huge firms such as Amazon, Netflix and the supermarkets to analyze your personal, individual preferences in order to suggest books, movies and foods you may like.

At first glance this may appear helpful but in reality it is only a sophisticated selling tool. This information-mining and consequent data has now become widespread through multiple industries. While the above firms are now gathering and entering your personal data, governments have already entered population health records into their national health databases, which could determine better policies.

The evidence that this "predictive modeling" for overall health policies can improve outcomes remains thin, however; it certainly has not been utilized at an individual level. Governments simply cannot afford to impose total population health schemes, let alone individualize them. However, as individuals, we are not so interested in health policies—we want the best individual advice for ourselves and family, which this data can now provide to protect us, prevent illness and improve our own health.

In fact, it would seem I am not the only one thinking this way. Statisticians, computer scientists and medics from the University of East Anglia are launching a new project to predict how long we will live. They will use "big data" to predict life expectancy—and to determine particularly how various chronic diseases and their treatments impact longevity.[12]

Theirs, however, is a 4-year project, whereas the data is already available to you in this book, which more importantly, advises how to avoid these illnesses. ***Live Longest*** is active preventive medicine you can start now.

Predictive Analysis – Health Forecasting

Predictive Analysis is the practice of extracting information from existing data sets in order to determine patterns and predict future outcomes and trends.

While to date, this approach has not been used for individual health care, the collected government data now provides age- and sex-specific, decade-by-decade lists that analyze what we prematurely or eventually die from or are disabled by. As Professor Dole observed, "Death in old age is inevitable but death before is not." There is no point pursuing what kills us when we are very old. What has to be identified are what causes are most likely to kill or disable us prematurely, and how we can identify these and prevent them. These lists allow for such individual Predictive Analysis or Health Forecasting of your immediate health risks.

Analyze, Predict and Prevent

We have all read about, or even know, ostensibly very fit and healthy people who suddenly have a premature heart attack, get cancer, suffer some fatal or debilitating illness or an "unlucky" accident at a relatively young age; then there are the hushed-up suicides or years of downtime due to depression or substance abuse.

But now there is a way to prevent or minimize most of these events. Now you can analyze, predict and prevent your age-related illness incidences and your health in its entirety, and not just illnesses after they occur.

Previous health plans and books have concentrated on lifestyle, diet, and exercise fads, or only treating illnesses after they occurred. There was no specific attempt to identify and avoid the illnesses we are *most likely* to encounter. It was as if diseases, illnesses and accidents never existed, and just gulping down a kale smoothie and multivitamins while performing hot yoga is enough. Or, if you are older, taking blood pressure tablets and statins is considered enough. But all these approaches simply ignore the facts of what illnesses or other conditions and accidents lurk for your age, and what you should really be doing to prevent these for your total, overall health.

Pigs Will Fly

In an article in *The Lancet* (one of the top 10 medical journals) the following laudable opinion was documented: "The responsibility for improving quality of life goes far beyond the health sector. Strategies are needed that better prevent and manage chronic conditions by extending affordable health care to all older adults."[13] The authors seem to hope that governments are going to find the money to fund their excellent suggestions; but history suggests otherwise. Their practical recommendations of low-cost disease prevention, early detection rather than treatment, and making better use of technology are exactly what should be done. But individuals will have to do this for themselves—as pigs will fly before governments could institute, let alone afford, such measures.

Preventive Medicine

Prevention definition: *"Approaches and activities aimed at reducing the likelihood that a disease or disorder will affect an individual, interrupting or slowing the progress of the disorder or reducing disability."* (The World Health Organization)[14]

Within this broad definition there are some more specific characterizations:

Primary prevention, which reduces the likelihood of developing a disease or disorder;

Secondary prevention, which interrupts, prevents or minimizes the progress of a disease or disorder at an early stage;

Tertiary prevention, which halts the progression of damage already done.

Our Greatest Health Concerns

The famous Mayo Clinic recently (2016) has done a decade-by-decade analysis of our greatest health concerns:

20s – healthy meal options

30s – maintaining healthy weight, parents' health issues

40s – maintaining healthy weight, children's health issues

50s–80s – their own health issues.

Evidence-Based Small, Pleasant, Acceptable Changes

In ***Live Longest***, first age-specific illnesses and accidents are identified; then the major evidence for *Successful Aging, Best Newtrition, Exercises* and *Weight Plans* is applied by substituting good for bad. One such example for nutrition is using olive oil instead of butter. Similar small, pleasant recommendations are made for successful aging, exercise and weight.

Little-Known "Gems" of Research That May Help (Much More Later)

Some recommended changes may appear small and trivial, but all have been researched and evidenced, with appropriate references. Each small bit of information can accumulate to contribute to your overall health and longevity. A sampling of such information and suggestions follows:

- *Get up and move: the least active people are 5 times more likely to die during the next 8 years than the most active.*
- *Infants do significantly better on developmental tests when their mothers consume more fruit during pregnancy.*
- *Swaddling is associated with double the risk for sudden infant death syndrome in the supine sleep position, and is even more dangerous in the side or prone position.*
- *The "Obesity Paradox": people who are overweight but not obese live longer—or do they?*
- *Meditation is linked to a 48% reduction in cardiovascular events.*
- *Chilies consumed almost every day resulted in a 14% lower risk of death.*
- *Driving fast or when upset increases risks by 13 and 10 times, respectively.*
- *Women who sunbathe are likely to live longer than those who avoid the sun, even though sunbathers are at an increased risk of developing skin cancer.*
- *Poor fitness levels in midlife are linked to brain shrinkage 20 years later.*
- *One soft drink/soda per day can increase the risk for type 2 diabetes by 26%, coronary heart disease by 35%, stroke by 16%.*
- *Energy drinks have been associated with sudden deaths.*
- *Regular tooth brushing may slow the progress of Alzheimer's disease, as may blueberries.*
- *Since WW2 there have been over 80,000 untested chemicals added to our food and environment.*

- *Eating meat may have kick-started the evolution of bigger brains, but cooked starchy foods (grains) together with more salivary amylase genes made us smarter still.*
- *Bus and tram users are slimmer than car drivers.*
- *Those who walked faster, or who walked seven blocks a day, had some 50% less coronary artery disease.*
- *Don't "self silence" during arguments (especially women: linked to 4 times more premature deaths).*
- *Premature mortality was reduced by 31% with 150, and 39% with 450 minutes/week of exercise.*
- *Fiber consumption reduced by > 55% between 1909 and 1975.*
- *Women who sat breakfast cereal out on their counters weighed 20 lbs more than those who didn't, and those with soft drinks sitting out weighed 24 to 26 lbs more. Those who had a fruit bowl weighed about 13 lbs less.*
- *Coffee more than halves the risk of type 2 diabetes and may reduce cancer of the colon by 26%.*
- *Most fruit drinks, juice and smoothies for UK kids have the entire daily recommended maximum intake of sugar.*
- *Daily fish oil offers no benefit for primary or secondary prevention of coronary heart disease, but fish does.*
- *Many synthetic vitamins are made from coal tar derivatives, chemically processed sugar, acids and industrial chemicals; with the word "natural" allowed to be used when only 10% of the content is natural.*
- *Vitamin C, in a multivitamin combination, did not reduce cardiovascular disease (CVD). However, when sourced from fruit and vegetables, it did.*
- *A 100 g portion of fruit per day was associated with one third less heart attacks and strokes.*
- *Those who ate the most fruit and vegetables had a 13% lower risk of CVD and a 20% lower risk of all-cause mortality compared with those who ate these foods only rarely.*
- *Vegetarians may have 40% more colorectal cancer than meat eaters but with lower diabetes, stroke & obesity.*
- *Daily consumption of sugar-sweetened drinks is linked to a higher incidence of biliary tract and gallbladder cancer.*
- *Taking beta-carotene, vitamin A and Vitamin E may increase mortality.*
- *There are 11 easily avoidable high-risk behaviors, yet 50% of our health problems, most cardiovascular disease and 90% of cancers are caused this way.*
- *There are only 13 vitamins we need, which are best available in food; but 83,000 health supplements are for sale.*

- *30 of the 31 "most commonly reported long-term conditions" can be treated.*
- *Mediterranean-MIND-DASH Diets are the basis for the best nutrition, as updated in* ***Live Longest Newtrition****.*
- *Just adding extra virgin olive oil (EVOO) and nuts can improve health.*
- *Breakfast is not an important meal; this was an advertising scam to sell bacon. Nor does it improve grades.*
- *There are an estimated 60 million type 2 diabetics in India. Most cases are attributed to an altered diet of processed foods.*
- *Having less than 20 teeth is associated with more dementia.*
- *Patients who consumed the most butter after a heart attack had 3 times the risk of dying within 42 months compared to those eating the Mediterranean Diet.*
- *In 2016, one's work schedule was considered as the top barrier to staying healthy.*
- *It is my suspicion that fit men under 50 who have a heart attack may be using cocaine, which is cardio-toxic.*
- *NSAIDS (anti-inflammatories) are cardio-toxic. If you have to take them, get the least toxic (Naprosyn).*
- *PPIs (proton pump inhibitors), now widely prescribed for stomach upsets, have been linked to Alzheimer's disease.*

I am not opposed to therapeutic drugs used correctly, but Big Pharma puts profits before people.

Men vs. Women

It has long been observed that women live longer than men, but the reasons why have not been clear. Humans are the only species in which one sex is known to have a survival advantage, and this sex difference in longevity may be one of the most robust features of human biology. The Human Mortality Database has complete lifespan tables for men and women from 38 countries that go back as far as 1751 for Sweden and 1816 for France; and for all 38 countries for every year in the database, female life expectancy at birth exceeds male life expectancy. The Gerontology Research Group data for the oldest of the old show that women make up 90% of the supercentenarians, those who live to 110 years of age or longer.

The birth cohorts are studied from the mid-1800s to the early 1900s for Iceland. This small, genetically homogenous country—which was beset by catastrophes such as famine, flooding, volcanic eruptions and disease epidemics—provides a particularly vivid example of female survival. Over that time, life expectancy at birth fell to as low as 21 years during catastrophes and rose to as high as 69 years during good times. Yet in every year, regardless of food availability or pestilence, women at the beginning of life and near its end survived better than men.[15]

A 2015 study found that vulnerability to heart disease is the biggest culprit behind a surge in higher death rates for men vs. women during the twentieth century. A review of global data points to heart disease as the culprit behind most of the excess deaths documented in adult men. Women are reaping the longevity benefits at a much faster rate, with a massive but uneven decrease in mortality. This uneven impact of cardiovascular illness-related deaths on men, especially during middle age and early older age, raises the question of whether men and women face different heart disease risks due to inherent biological risks and/or protective factors at different points in their lives.[16] The prognosis for women with heart disease, however, is often worse, as they have narrower coronary arteries. And recently this gap between men and women's survival has narrowed as women smoke and drink more and work longer hours. And for all their robustness relative to men in terms of survival, women on average appear to be in poorer health than men through adult life. This higher prevalence of physical limitations in later life is seen not only in Western societies, the data shows, but also for women in Bangladesh, China, Egypt, Guatemala, India, Indonesia, Jamaica, Malaysia, Mexico, the Philippines, Thailand and Tunisia. [17] Women who worked over 60 hours a week over three decades triple their risk for diabetes, heart trouble and arthritis. The increased risks begin after 40 hrs a week.[18] Live Longest advice is for both sexes and the lists highlight the different illnesses for each.

But Wait! There's More!

It is not only heart attacks which can now be prevented, but most of the top 10 (or even 20) fatal or debilitating illnesses specific to your age. Now by reviewing the lists of the Causes of Death and Disabilities, the top 10 illnesses can be analyzed. Now there can be far fewer young widows or widowers.

And Yet More: Urine Analysis Could Help To Slow Age-Related Diseases

Humans age in two different ways. Normal aging, also known as primary aging, is the result of cellular processes, which lead to physiological changes as people get older. This process occurs naturally without the influence of disease, and currently limits the maximum human lifespan to around 120 years. Pathologic, or secondary, aging is caused by internal processes, which shorten lifespan through disease or the side effects of an unhealthy lifestyle.

Now research has found differences between "normal" aging and pathologic aging at the molecular level in urine samples, using a process known as *proteome analysis*. This is a new research method which detects changes in the body by analyzing specific protein and common age-correlated peptide patterns. It is thought that early therapy may help to avoid or slow down the emergence of age-related diseases and, as a consequence, slow down secondary aging in humans. Tests have already shown the beneficial effects of including as little as 20 ml of olive oil in the diet each day. Reduction in the biomarker for coronary heart disease reduced after only six weeks.[19]

Aging processes include chronic low-grade inflammation not related to infection, degradation of cells, molecular (DNA, proteins, sugars) damage / failure of stem cells and progenitor cell functions.

A workshop entitled "Interventions to Slow Aging in Humans: Are We Ready?"[20] was held in Erice, Italy, on October 8–13, 2013, to bring together leading experts in the biology and genetics of aging and obtain a consensus related to the discovery and development of safe interventions to slow aging and increase healthy lifespan in humans.There was consensus that there is sufficient evidence that aging interventions will delay and prevent disease onset for many chronic conditions of adult and old age. Essential pathways have been identified, and behavioral, dietary, and pharmacologic approaches have emerged. These were:

(i) dietary interventions mimicking chronic dietary restriction (periodic fasting-mimicking diets, protein restriction, etc.);

(ii) drugs that inhibit the growth hormone/IGF-I axis;

(iii) drugs that inhibit the mTOR–S6K pathway; or

(iv) drugs that activate AMPK or specific sirtuins.

These choices were based in part on consistent evidence for the prolongevity effects and ability of these interventions to prevent or delay multiple age-related diseases and improve healthspan in simple model organisms and rodents and their potential to be safe and effective in extending human healthspan.

Laron's syndrome, or Laron-type dwarfism, is an autosomal recessive disorder characterized by an insensitivity to growth hormone (GH), usually caused by a mutant growth hormone receptor. Apart from their dwarfism, these patients don't age and don't suffer from cancer or diabetes. An extract from them has been made into a drug, Rapamycin, which has been shown to extend life in mice. Thirty-three percent of these people live in Equador where the Longevity Center of Los Angeles is doing research.

A group of experts on aging, university scientists joined together by the American Federation for Aging Research and who call themselves "geroscientists," are investigating one or more drugs that can slow the rate of aging and the development of the costly, debilitating chronic ailments that typically accompany it. The geroscientists will target the processes fundamental to aging that underlie all age-related chronic diseases: chronic low-grade inflammation unrelated to infection; cellular degradation; damage to major molecules like DNA, proteins and sugars; and failure of stem cells and other progenitor cells to function properly. They will test the drug metformin in a placebo-controlled trial involving 3,000 elderly people to see if it will delay the development or progression of a variety of age-related ailments, including heart disease, cancer and dementia. Rapamycin, an immune modulator used in organ transplantation, has been the most effective to date.

Death-Defying Future Ventures

Looking to the future, there are moves afoot to prolong life past its present limits. Currently the Japanese live longest, into their mid-80s, while Americans have the most individuals in the top 100 oldest people. Prolonging life past these present "normal" limits will, however, be very expensive. Enter a new breed of Silicon Valley entrepreneurs with big resources at their disposal. According to some gerontologists we are headed toward a 1% phenomenon, with only the very wealthy able to afford the cutting-edge healthcare that adds meaningfully to life. Predicted breakthroughs in the next 15 or 20 years will have to do with aging itself—actually stopping the biological clock. *The Week* magazine's headline summed it up: "How Silicon Valley's billionaires are trying to defy death." The new research money is largely private and unregulated. The big breakthroughs will be very expensive and available only to the very wealthy, at least initially. Craig Venter, one of the first scientists to sequence the human genome, launched a company in 2014 called Human Longevity Inc. that plans to apply genetic sequencing to some of the most challenging issues involving aging. Google Inc. launched Calico, a company focused on extending lifespans, in 2013. There is also big money chasing longevity from Facebook Inc., eBay Inc. and Napster fortunes.

The Near Future

Don't hold your breath: by "near" I mean at least 10 years. But there are some exciting, promising breakthroughs, the latest of which is an anti-cancer vaccine developed in Germany. What they did was to identify all the "markers" on cancer cells and then develop a vaccine against them. While the research was done on mice, it would seem eminently transferable to humans to prevent all cancers; and the vaccine would continue to circulate in our bodies such that permanent immunity is provided.

Another advance is the decoding and understanding of the human genome, which has allowed analysis of mutations to individual genes that cause infections, inflammation, cancer and neurodegenerative diseases. The next step will be to learn how to turn off, rather than turn on, these mutations.

In summary, substantial attempts to extend our health span through more emphasis on fitness and prevention are coinciding with breakthroughs in pharmaceuticals, stem cell therapies, immuno-vaccines and genetic manipulation; but the fruits of these advances are years, if not decades, away. While all this is potentially exciting, what can be done now, and mostly without expense, can be identified with the information of Predictive Analysis, combined with with age-specific data on the diseases most likely to affect us and, most importantly, how to prevent them.

Dietary Supplements

Fascinating Canadian research on plant extracts (PEs) has found six which would seem to slow the aging process in a combination of ways. This research, however, was done on yeast, as the aging metabolic pathways of yeast are similar to those of humans. The challenge for the future is to assess whether any of the six PEs can delay the onset and progression of chronic diseases associated with human aging. Among such diseases are arthritis, diabetes, heart disease, kidney disease, liver dysfunction, sarcopenia, stroke, neurodegenerative diseases (including Parkinson's, Alzheimer's and Huntington's diseases), and many forms of cancer. Several features of the six PEs represent potential interventions for decelerating chronic diseases of old age:

1) The six PEs are caloric restriction (CR) mimetics that imitate the aging-delaying effects of the CR diet in yeast under non-CR conditions; 2) they are geroprotectors that slow yeast aging by eliciting a hormetic stress response; 3) they extend yeast longevity more efficiently than any lifespan-prolonging chemical compound yet described; 4) they delay aging through signaling pathways and protein kinases implicated in such age-related pathologies as type 2 diabetes, neurodegenerative diseases, cardiac hypertrophy, cardiovascular disease, sarcopenia and cancers; and 5) they extend longevity and delay the onset of age-related diseases in other eukaryotic model organisms. The potential of using the six aging-delaying PEs for delaying the onset of age-related diseases in humans is further underscored by the fact that the Health Canada government agency classifies these PEs as safe for human consumption and recommends using five of them as health-improving supplements with clinically proven benefits to human health :

The PEs:

1. Black Cohosh Cimicifuga or Actaea racemosa 0.5% (w/v)
2. Valerian Valeriana officinalis L. 0.5% (w/v)
3. Purple Passion flower Passiflora incarnata L. 1.0% (w/v)
4. Ginkgo biloba, 0.1% (w/v) 0.3% (w/v)
5. Celery Apium graveolens L. and 0.1% (w/v)
6. White Willow Barkfrom Salix alba

Each of the six PEs delays aging through different signaling pathways and/or protein kinases; this study also revealed that certain combinations markedly increase aging-delaying proficiencies of each other. Furthermore, all combinations display additive or synergistic effects on the extent of aging delay. It is known that the network of longevity-defining signaling pathways/ protein kinases is controlled by such aging-delaying chemical compounds as resveratrol, rapamycin, caffeine, spermidine, myriocin, methionine sulfoxide, lithocholic acid and cryptotanshinone.

Author's Comment:

This research ("Six plant extracts delay yeast chronological aging through different signaling pathways[2]," was a well-conducted study, with plant extracts exquisitely refined and diluted to exact concentrations and then combined to deliver this impressive result. These scientists or their university have apparently patented their formula. Just rushing out and buying these supplements will not reproduce their formula. That said, however, as they point out, Health Canada already recommends five of these six and they are readily available. *Salix alba*—white willow bark—seemed the most potent, but they all work along different pathways, hence the greater effect when combined.

However, before taking them, if you are on any medications , pregnant or breast feeding. you should check for any interactions.

Willow bark was the origin of aspirin, which, if taken for long enough, seems to reduce the incidence of cancer of the colon (CAC); it is also an anti-coagulant and people on anticoagulants must consult their doctor. Purple Passion Flower also seems to have anticoagulant properties, and the Mayo clinic advises against its use in pregnancy. Gingko is also an anticoagulant. Black Cohosh has been occasionally associated with liver failure. Valerian can have side effects.

Play the Percentages and Odds

Knowing the odds against us allows us to best respond to even up those odds. While this may sound obvious, in health it is not. The high-risk behaviors responsible for an estimated 50% or more of our premature demise or disabilities include some quite surprising behaviors we often take for granted. By knowing these risk factors along with the prevalence, incidence and specific-age-related illnesses, we can reduce the odds.

We understand that reducing the odds against us offers us the greatest chance of success when it comes to sports and games. We know that "backing the long shot" is just that; it does not offer the best odds. Having played tennis against Wimbledon, US and French Champions who kindly let me occasionally hit the ball back, I quickly learned how much, even against an inept opponent like myself, they play the percentage game, and thereby reduce the odds. They know which shot has the greatest chance of success. The center of the net is some six inches lower than the outside net on the singles lines, so where do they

---

[2] Oncotarget, *July 18, 2016,* doi: 10.18632/oncotarget.10689)

hit most shots? Across the center. It is lower; it offers a greater percentage for success. Knowing the odds, they do not make high-risk shots. The same principle applies with world championship poker or any other competitive venture.

To win at health, we also have to know the odds and play the percentages. What are the odds of a heart attack at your age? What are the odds of depression? If one illness occurs 70% more than others at your age, you can improve your chances by knowing how to avoid it. Most people, including my doctor colleagues, don't know the exact odds that would improve their patients' health.

When it comes to health we seemingly blunder on, following disproven rituals such as the "annual check-up or physical," which is tantamount to blindly playing cards without knowing the rules, or going for a backhand down the line which only has a 15% chance compared with a forehand across the middle of the net at 90% success. What are the odds (the rate of occurrence) for a 40-year-old woman to get breast cancer? Are they more or less than her odds of having a heart attack, depression, suicide, and diabetes? If the chances are greater, would it not make sense to concentrate on this instead of the 360-to-1 option? Yet many of us do the latter because we don't know the age-rates and order in which illnesses occur.

At best, we buy vitamins and supplements (very bad odds), follow some fad diet (bad odds), exercise incorrectly (well, at least it's exercise, but there are now better methods) and get an annual check-up from our doctor which all health authorities now recognize as being not very effective (not good odds but at least it may pick up something). Then, out of the blue, to our complete surprise because we are so super-fit and health-nutty, we get struck down with an illness which, had we known what to look out for, we may well have prevented.

Or, at worst, we eat the wrong foods, don't exercise, don't get checked, and get heart disease, blood pressure, have a disabling stroke, get diabetes, have to gobble down 17 drugs a day in a nursing home while wearing diapers, and die 20 years before we should.

This need not be.

If we know what illnesses are most likely, we can take specific and long-term preventive measures. ***Live Longest*** identifies these illnesses for each sex and each age group and then provides the best and latest evidenced and documented preventive advice as to Prediction, Early Diagnosis, Successful Aging, Nutrition, Weight, and Exercise.

Live Longest - Missing Keys Approach

The Easy Changes to Individual Better Health and Longer Life

1. Death and Disability Lists: Predictive Analysis – Health Forecasting

Massive national data as to what illnesses occur at what age for either sex has been recorded. This then provides for Predictive Analysis, which allows for more relevant focus on those specific serious illnesses *you* are most likely to now encounter, and optimizes preventive stratagems or diagnosing illnesses when they are curable.

2. Specific Preventive Practices – Latest Information

The evidence from new trials has revealed more refined improvements in how to prevent most of the illnesses that prematurely kill or debilitate us. For example, our greatest killer is cardiovascular disease, but wonderfully pleasant foods can prevent much of it. Many cancers are preventable.

3. Complete Health Plan - The Live Longest Series.

8. Who Lives the Longest

The Blue Zones:

Blue Zones was coined to identify a demographic or geographic area where people live longer and evolved when demographers drew concentric blue circles on a map of villages in Sardinia's Nuoro province with the highest concentration of male centenarians. [3]

Five regions were identified in Buettner's book *The Blue Zones: Lessons for Living Longer from People Who've Lived the Longest*:

1. ***Sardinia*, *Italy*** (particularly Ogliastra, Barbagia di Ollolai and Barbagia of Seulo): one team of demographers found a hot spot of longevity in mountain villages where an amazing proportion of men reach the age of 100 years. In particular, a village located in the Barbagia of Seulo, holds the record of 20 centenarians from 1996 to 2016, that confirms it is " the place where people live the longest in the world "[

2. ***Okinawa*, *Japan:*** another team examined a group that is among the longest-lived on Earth.

3. ***Loma Linda, California***: Seventh-day Adventists

4. ***Nicoya Peninsula, Costa Rica:*** A peninsula of long living men

5. ***Ikaria, Greece:*** has the highest percentage of 90-year-olds on the planet – nearly 1 out of 3 people make it to their 90s. Ikarians have about 20 percent lower rates of cancer, 50 percent lower rates of heart disease and almost no dementia.

6. ***Öland, Sweden*** - southern Småland and northeastern Skåne,

7. ***Acciaroli, Italy:*** one-third of its citizens (~ 300 persons) live at least 80 years.

Some earlier studies had identified **Abkhazia, Caucasia, Vilicanba, Ecuador** and the **Hunza Valley, Pakistan** as places where people also lived longer but these have been debunked as

---

[3] "Identification of a geographic area characterized by extreme longevity in the Sardinia island: the AKEA study". *Experimental Gerontology.* **39** (9): 1423–1429. doi:10.1016/j.exger.2004.06.016.

there were no reliable records and the elderly were prone to exaggerate their age. Nevertheless their physical lifestyle, primitive plant based diet and social integration are similar to the above and maybe some are living longer.

Individual Longevity Top 100:

The USA: 50

Japan: 19

UK: 8

France: 6

Spain: 3

Italy: 2

Australia: 1

National Life Expectancy Top 10 Countries:

2013 (WHO)	*2015*
1. Japan	1. Monaco
2. Andorra	2. Japan
3. Singapore	3. Singapore
4. Hong Kong	4. Macau
5. San Marino	5. San Marino
6. Iceland	6. Iceland
7. Italy	7. Hong Kong
8. Sweden	8. Andorra
9. Australia	9. Switzerland
10. Switzerland	10. Guernsey

People Who Live The Longest:

1. The Rich
2. Intelligence and Genetics
3. The Blue Zones
4. Seventh Day Adventists of California
5. Individuals 6. Nations

1. The Rich

The rich live longer than the poor, with an ever widening dichotomy. Despite significant advances in medicine and technology, the longevity gap between high-income (socioeconomic classes 1 and 2) and low-income groups (socioeconomic groups 4 and 5) has been increasing sharply. In 2016 economists at the Brookings Institution found that the difference in life span after age 50, between richest and poorest, has more than doubled since the 1970s.

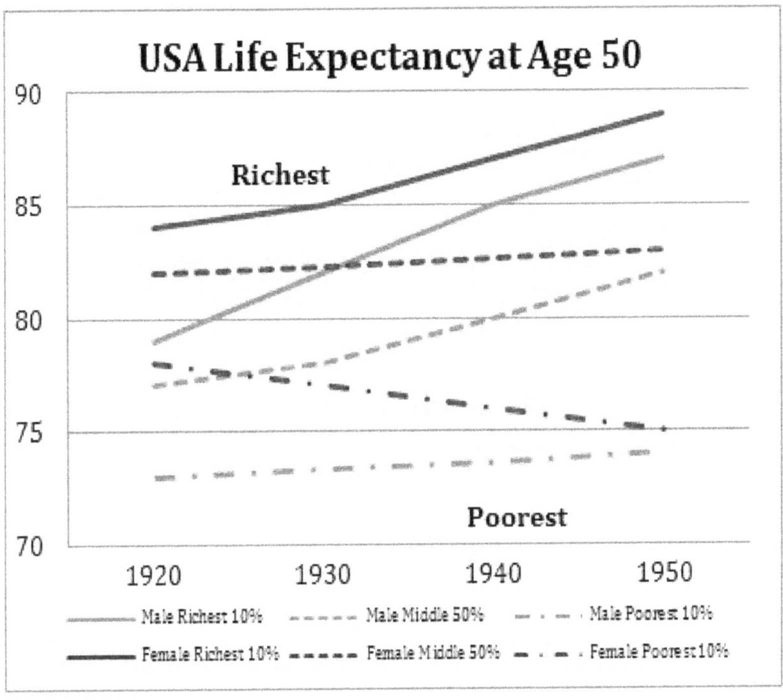

Based on U. of Michigan Health and Retirement

In the United Kingdom, between 1930 and 1990, despite the best medical treatments, tests, investigations, medicines, hospitals and operations being offered and supplied *for free,* from the late 1940s, the unskilled classes' health has become nearly 3 times worse than the health of the more affluent professional class. Access to free medical care does not, by itself, help you live longer. You need this new evidence, information and advice.

A 2016 *JAMA* study provides a comprehensive look at income and life expectancy in the United States.[21] Using federal income tax and Social Security data from 1999 to 2014, researchers estimated mortality rates and calculated period life expectancy based on participants' taxable household income at age 40. Based on 1.4 billion person-years of data, researchers concluded:

Life expectancy increased continuously with household income. The discrepancy in life expectancy increased from 2001 to 2014: people in the top 5% of income increased their life expectancy by as much as 3 years, while the bottom 5% saw little change. Differences in lifespan were most pronounced in comparisons of the extremely wealthy and extremely poor. Compared with the bottom 1% of income distribution, men in the top 1% lived nearly 15 years longer, while women lived 10 years longer—a gap equivalent to the effect of a lifetime of smoking.

Most of the variation in life expectancies observed across geographic areas was tied to differences in health behaviors, not healthcare access or other factors.[22] Those in the low socioeconomic group suffered medical causes of death such as heart disease and cancer, after exhibiting obesity and behaviors such as higher rates of smoking and less exercise. These intrinsic causes were more prevalent than external causes such as car crashes, suicide, homicide or lack of access to health care.

The conclusion is that the low socioeconomic groups do not look after themselves as well as the higher socioeconomic groups. This at least is the United Kingdom experience (see chart below), where free hospitals and medical treatments did not improve their lot, rather it became worse over time.

It would seem to the author that the first step to improve this situation is evidenced health education. Learning about nutrition, exercise and high-risk behavior should be made compulsory in schools. The information would, however, have to be enthusiastically, properly and repetitively presented, with all junk foods banned from school cafeterias and canteens—which currently are often subsidized by the fast-food industry, such that these outlets then come to depend on the industry to exist. The lower socioeconomic groups most often simply don't know what is good or bad food.

Smoking has been reduced by such aggressive educational programs. The next step would be the subsidized provision of a piece of fruit a day—substituting good for bad while condemning the bad and talking up the benefits of the good.

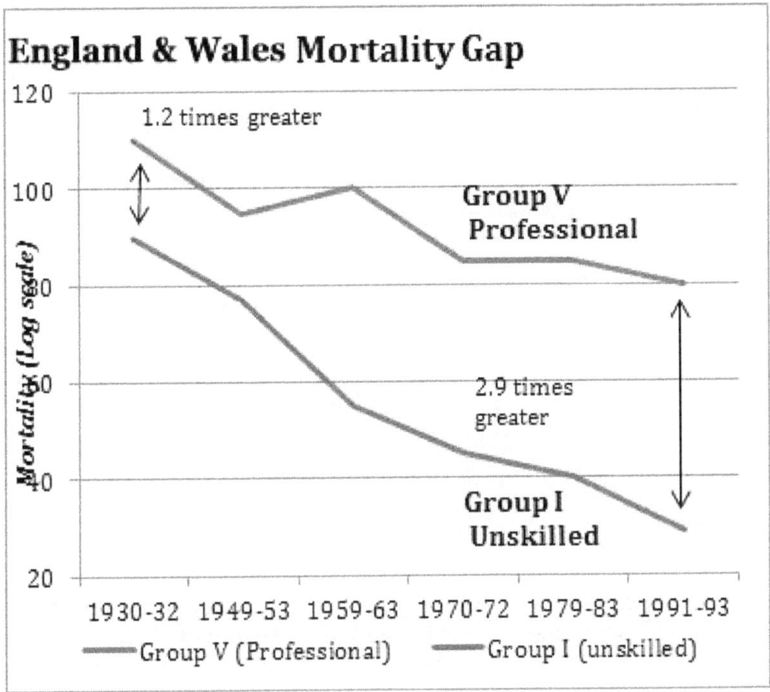

Office for National Statistics

2. Intelligence and Genetics

A study in 2015 analyzed the causes of the link between intelligence and longer lifespan. It noted that many previous studies have found this correlation, but distinguishing the cause of the relationship is difficult. Common causes posited include socioeconomic status affecting intelligence and life expectancy, higher intelligence causing more healthy behavior choices, and shared genetic factors influencing both intelligence and health. By analyzing three data sets of twins from the United States, Sweden and Denmark, the researchers determined that genetics contributed the most to the correlation between lifespan and intelligence.

3. The Blue Zones

Intelligence is not necessary in the Blue Zones. These are characterized by a “primitive” fresh produce diet with little meat, hard physical activity and good social integration.

4. Seventh-Day Adventists (of California)

On average Adventist men live 7.3 years longer and Adventist women live 4.4 years longer than other Californians.

Five simple health behaviors promoted by the Seventh-day Adventist Church for more than 100 years (not smoking, eating a plant-based diet, eating nuts several times per week, regular exercise and maintaining normal body weight) increase life span up to 10 years.

5. Individuals

It is intriguing that, while the United States is overall poor for longevity, it has by far the greatest number of longest-living individuals of any nation. One can only assume they are benefitting from access to the world's best and latest medical advice and care.

6. Nations

As a nation, the Japanese live longest. This is thought to be because of their predominantly fish and seaweed diet. However, the Okinawans, some of the longest living people, swear by purple sweet potato (eating up to 0.5kg a day).

While the United States has more longer-living *individuals* than any other nationality, the combined national average for the whole general population is way down in the mid-30s for longevity. And while it may be thought that compromised access to hospitals and health care plays a major part in the premature deaths of the poor, limited access to health care accounts for surprisingly few premature deaths in America.

Different sources provide slightly different lists, which may account for some differences. It is extremely difficult to draw any conclusions except that Japan, with its traditional diet, and Iceland, with its pristine environment, are always in the top 10. But Hong Kong, Singapore and now Monaco are listed, three of the most densely populated places on earth. San Marino is a mountainous microstate surrounded by Italy, so in effect it is Italian for these purposes. Switzerland is also right up there. We might surmise that stable government provides security and less stress, and should therefore be conducive to longevity, but Hong Kong and Italy don't seem to provide it and make the list anyway.

Living Longer

Living healthy and well until we are 85 would seem a reasonable objective and expectation, but a health advisor to the president of the United States has written how he "hopes to die at 75" due to the deteriorations that seem to overwhelm us at that age. However, a quick look at *The New York Times* or the *London Daily Telegraph*'s obituaries soon shows a great number of vital people dying well beyond 75.

The health information here offers unique, hitherto unused official data, now collated into one plan for the first time, as to how we should all live healthy and vital well beyond 75.

The Bad News

Even though both sexes are living longer, women's life expectancy—Healthy Life Expectancy (HLE), the length of time they would typically expect to live in full health—has decreased. This trend is thought to be caused by women adopting high-risk behaviors of men such as smoking, drinking and working longer hours.[23]

To Live Longer, Money or Education Is Not Absolutely Necessary – But the Correct Information Is

So what is the cause of disparities in longevity, and how can we live as long as the rich? The examples of the Japanese, the Californian Adventists and the Blue Zones of the world, where people live longest, would suggest that money is not the answer. It is their environment, lifestyle, nutrition and activities, which optimize the conditions for longevity. While we can to a large extent mimic these conditions, the affluent West, with its processed foods, cars, and stressful long hours of work, has introduced new illnesses that cause premature deaths. In the West cardiovascular disease is our greatest killer, but it is relatively unknown in Japan or the Blue Zones, as are our next greatest killers, breast, prostate and colon cancer. Even if we try to mimic the Blue Zone or Japanese ways with diet and exercise, our Western way of life is so pervasive that still we are struck down with unexpected "Western" illnesses but the Adventists in California seem to be able to avoid it.

If we know what these illnesses are and when they are most likely to strike us, then we can take specific measures to avoid or minimize them. This is the Missing Key, to go along with the usual health advice suggesting good diet, exercise, keeping trim and not smoking. But do you want to live past 75?

This book on Predictive Health Forecasting allows for earlier Health Risk Identification and therefore better-focused, complete Prevention Plans for Successful Aging, Lifestyle, Nutrition, Exercise and Weight.

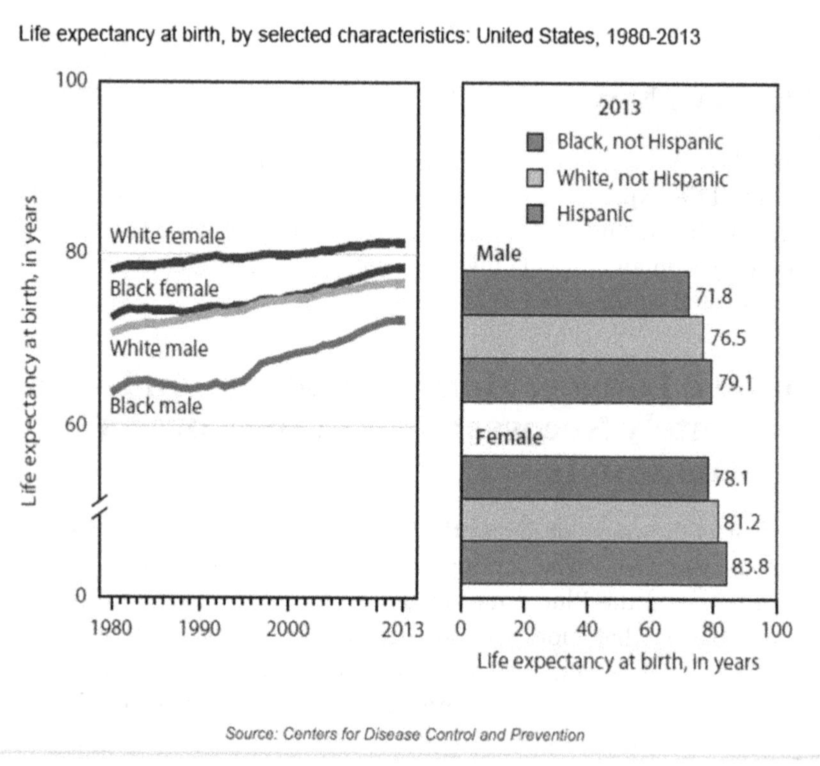

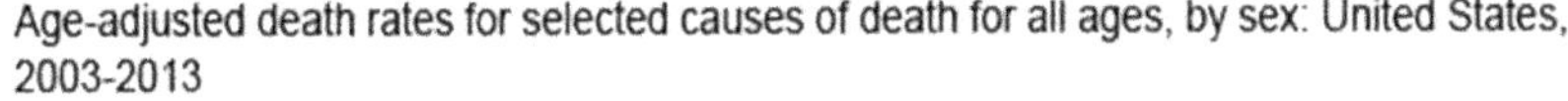

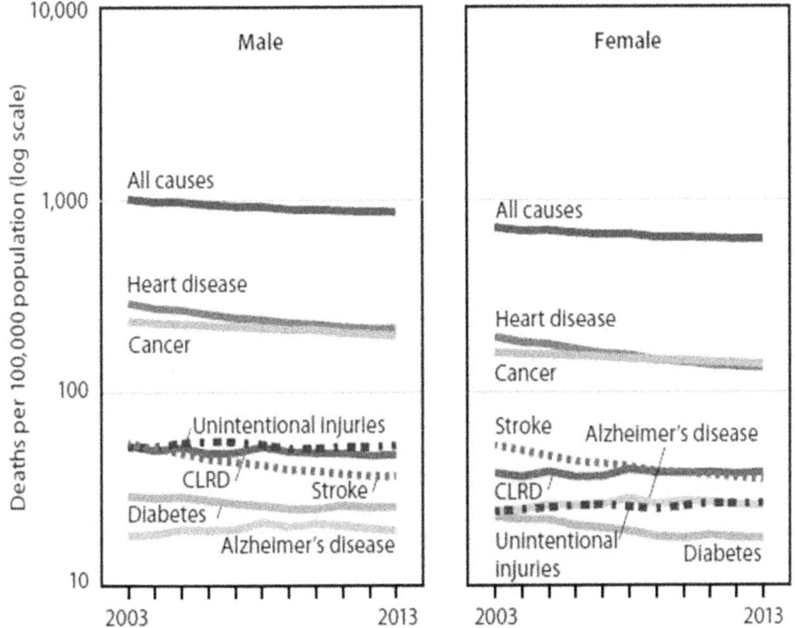

"> *Source: Centers for Disease Control and Prevention*

Whereas in 1999, cardiovascular disease (CVD) excluding stroke was the main cause of death in all US states except Alaska, 14 years later, deaths from cancer surpassed those from CVD in almost half of the states, a newer study reports.[58]

About half of the dramatic reduction in heart-disease mortality can be attributed to better treatments such as revascularization and about half to reductions in risk factors such as smoking, cholesterol, and blood pressure, but not BMI or diabetes.[59]

The Hispanic Paradox: Latinos Age at a Slower Rate

According to the Centers for Disease Control and Prevention, Latinos in the United States live an average of three years longer than Caucasians, with a life expectancy of 82 versus 79. At any age, healthy Latino adults face a 30% lower risk of death than other racial groups (two African groups, African-Americans, Caucasians, East Asians, Latinos and an indigenous people who are genetically related to Latinos, the Tsimane of Bolivia), who aged even slower with minimal signs and very little evidence of the chronic diseases that commonly afflict modern society such as heart disease, diabetes, hypertension, obesity or clogged arteries, despite frequent infections.

The research also found that men's blood and brain tissue ages faster than women's from the same ethnic groups. The discovery could explain why women have a higher life expectancy than men.[60]

Poor Lifestyles Lose Canadians Six Years of Life

Smoking, poor diet, physical inactivity, and unhealthy alcohol consumption contribute to about 50% of deaths in Canada and are costing an estimated six years of life.

Research found:

- 26% of all deaths are attributable to smoking.
- 24% of all deaths are attributable to physical inactivity.
- 12% of all deaths are attributable to poor diet.
- 0.4% of all deaths are attributable to unhealthy alcohol consumption.

For men, smoking was the top risk factor, representing a loss of 3.1 years. For women it was lack of physical activity, representing a loss of 3 years.

Canadians who followed recommended healthy behaviors had a life expectancy 17.9 years greater than individuals with the unhealthiest behaviours.[61]

Keep Your Friends Closer But Your Family Closer

Older individuals who have more family in their network, as well as older people who are closer with their family, are less likely to die; no such associations were observed for number of or closeness to friends. But those who listed more non-spousal family members in their network—irrespective of closeness—had lower odds of death compared to those who listed fewer family members.[63]

Twins, Especially Male Identical Twins, Live Longer

It is thought this reflects the benefits of lifelong social support. The lifespan was extended more for identical rather than fraternal twins, which may reflect the strength of the social bond.[64]

9. "I Hope to Die At 75"

Doctors Disagree

In October 2014, Dr Ezekiel Emanuel, one of the chief architects of US President Obama's Affordable Care Act, unleashed controversy after he published an article in the *Atlantic* magazine entitled, "Why I hope to die at 75."[24] He wrote about the problems of aging beyond 75, including a sharp drop-off in creativity, functional declines, reduced mental capacity and burdens on family members. He wrote that while death is a loss, "living too long is also a loss," and concluded, "Seventy-five. That's all I want to live."

His comments triggered an outpouring of mostly anger at the *Atlantic* website, where over 4000 responses were posted. Many echoed Archer R. Gravely, who wrote, inter alia, "I certainly have no desire to 'live' at an advanced age in a nursing home but I know a number of 80+ folks who have a pretty good time going fishing and shooting at the range."

Emanuel said that once he is 75, he will not actively end his life but he "won't try to prolong it, either." He said that the default position of doctors is "almost invariably" to order tests and treatments. But Emanuel prefers to "flip... this default on its head," writing that he takes guidance from William Osler, who wrote in his textbook, *The Principles and Practice of Medicine*: "Pneumonia may well be called the friend of the aged" and that by dying of "an acute, short, not often painful illness, the old man escapes those 'cold gradations of decay' so distressing to himself and to his friends." Emanuel, a bioethicist and oncologist (cancer specialist), described his "Osler-inspired philosophy" by saying that at 75 and beyond he will "stop getting any regular preventive tests, screenings or interventions. I will accept only palliative—not curative—treatments if I am suffering pain or other disability."

I must say that I find his assertion that he will not accept "curative treatments" rather odd, if that is actually, as reported, what he said. Run that past me again? I too have devoured Sir William Osler's Principles and put them into practice and I simply can't agree that Osler would withhold curative treatments to those mentally intact and otherwise physically able. I have diagnosed and excised otherwise fatal cancers in over-75-year old patients who are now cured, living and functioning well more than 10 years later. If one of these were Dr Emanuel, is he saying he would not want me to excise the cancer but would prefer to let it go to metastasize to his liver and brain, and to die a horrible death? And would he want me, in the condition described below, to endure incredible pain and lose the use of my legs while only taking palliation in the form of soporofic, addictive pain killers, when an elegant operation would prove curative, restoring full, pain-free function?

75 and Still Going Strong

By unfortunate coincidence or serendipity, when I started the formal writing of this book in 2015 (though the actual research goes back over 50 years) I wrote how I was "actually rapidly approaching my 75th birthday, still find my wife disturbingly attractive, work 10 hours a day, by choice, in my busy solo medical clinic doing quite delicate facial operations. I am in good health with normal blood pressure and cholesterol, take no medication (except an occasional paracetamol/acetaminophen for a hangover), have just completed two medical textbooks of some 1,000 pages and have intensively studied, for many years, how to prevent premature death and disabilities. As such, somewhat immodestly I seem to have personally demonstrated that it actually is possible to live longer, be healthy, even productive, and with an excellent quality of life past 75. And how to do this is now available to everyone. You don't really need money, just the right information and the motivation, which, if you've read this far, you have.

A year later, I am now 75; and while a few things have changed, most haven't. I have no intention, nor do I hope, to die this year. I could say "fingers crossed" but instead I prefer to access the latest medical information, techniques and improvements. As to not accepting curative treatments, as Dr Emanuel says he will not do at 75, I had to face some inevitable consequences of getting old, and back surgery was one of them. While it was not life-threatening, it certainly was Quality of Life threatening. I had a low opinion of back surgery, which was reinforced when I examined an American orthopedic surgeon just a few months prior, who most strongly advised me "to avoid it." His operation had been a wretched failure; and when my own surgeon asked bemusedly "why I had waited so long" I answered that it was "because I knew a lot about back surgery." He laughed and assured me "things have changed." And they had. I have lived long enough to see back surgery emerge from the primeval swamp of barbaric butchery to elegant microsurgery. It was unavoidable in my case (spinal stenosis—a narrowing of the spinal canal with compression of the spinal cord and spondylolethiasis—where one vertebra moves forward to further compress the spinal cord). The operation was curative and I returned to work in less than four weeks. I am not boasting or being brave: the Surgeon did a great job! The newly designed titanium screws also bring yet more improvements. I only cite this event as a firsthand experience that would seem to completely contradict Dr Emanuel's disdain for such curative interventions.

More Good News

And the whole of medicine is rocketing ahead with such wonderful and incredible advances... if you know how to access them. Even so, the better you look after yourself *now*, any such interventions are minimized and your recovery maximized. That said, there are, like greying hair, some inescapable imposts of age; but, as with my back, most are fixable. The progress of modern medicine is incredible and can only get better.

Morbid Personalities and Prophets of Doom

Dr Emanuel was only 57 years old in 2014 when he wanted to die at 75. I saw a photo of him in 2016; he is a good-looking man radiating confidence and health. In his specialty of treating cancer, he would mostly see patients with established, incurable diseases, already too late to effect a cure. Treating the incurable is a laudable but morbid specialty, which surely must influence one's outlook. I would like to get his later opinion, based on his own longer experience and personal realizations, or insights, if and when he is 75 years old. I not only absolutely refute his death wish ultimatum but also now provide the information that allows us to live well past 75.

Nevertheless

Dr Emanuel's choice of 75 is not altogether curious or even totally wrong (even though I offer what I feel is a viable alternative) because, while today's 75 "is the new 65," nevertheless our health symptoms seem to suddenly deteriorate at age 75. The chapter "Life Begins at 40" shows how our asymptomatic parameters of health (changes we mostly don't notice, which are just biochemical or only visible by x-rays) at age 75 become symptomatic and we "suddenly" deteriorate. Joints give out, blood pressure and heart troubles intervene, eyesight and hearing deteriorate and yes, even our recollection of words may suggest we are not as sharp. The indignities and the horrors of old age now confront us. Most of us do not want to then live as a progressively debilitated nursing home resident undergoing Osler's "cold gradations of decay."

But, Then Again, to Look on the Bright Side

Most of the old-age imposts are eminently treatable. At 104 years old Edith Varley had a hip replacement; her "terrible pain," according to her daughter, has been relieved and she is now able to walk with a frame. But the oldest such patient was Gladys Hooper, 112 years old when she had her operation in 2015 at St Mary's hospital, Newport, UK.

Like all of us, I wish to live longer while enjoying good to moderate health, which is now possible. It was reported in the prestigious *Archives of Internal Medicine* that, after following some 1,000 men, the probability of a 90-year life span at age 70 years was 54% in the absence of smoking, diabetes, obesity, hypertension, or sedentary lifestyle. More than 68% of those rated their late-life health as excellent or very good; they had a lower incidence of chronic diseases, and were 3 to 5 years older at disease onset. The 2015 report from the International Longevity Centre-UK reveals that the elderly are much healthier than just a decade ago. Serious illnesses in those over 50 had dropped by some 2% in just a decade, and that figure was 6% for those 65 to 69. American men live an average of 2 years longer than they did in 2000, and women have an additional 2.4 years, according to mortality projections released in 2014 by the Society of Actuaries. Along with the gender gap, higher-income white-collar workers outlive blue-collar workers by 2.5 years, on average, from age 65. Other research points to a sizable longevity gap by educational attainment and race as well as income, as pointed out in chapter 8.

There has been a significant recent improvement in health such that people are living well until their 80s—certainly if they have a high income and education. If these advances continue, improvements in health can be reasonably expected when over 80. And if good habits and lifestyles are adopted, let alone early identification of potential problems, living to 80+ with "excellent or very good" health (as above) may well be possible. If 75 were the new 65, then 85 would seem achievable as the new 75.

The Real Imposts of Age

The more educated access better health information and can afford better food, but the world's longest-living people, in the Blue Zones (section 6, in Book 2) are invariably poor and uneducated peasants. So money isn't necessary for their longevity. Their conditions enforce a healthy lifestyle, which is analyzed in Book 3. But there is danger ahead for the rich and educated people, who are ostensibly living a healthy lifestyle, because in an affluent society they are increasingly struck down prematurely by the new "Diseases of Affluence."

Today as we age and live longer, new illnesses intrude. One such illness is a potential epidemic but may be asymptomatic. Silent atrial fibrillation and other similar heart arrhythmias are potentially fatal but also fairly easily treated. If not treated the person nearly certainly will have a stroke or slide into heart failure. The person either dies a sudden death, is left a semi-paralyzed cripple or slowly suffocates to death—when it is treatable and preventable! It is now recommended that anyone over 65 should have an annual ECG/EKG, as this test enables the diagnosis. Prime Minister Tony Blair was diagnosed in 2003 with supraventricular tachycardia (SVT), a different type of arrhythmia than atrial fibrillation (AF). He was treated with cardio version and eventually underwent catheter ablation to restore his heart's natural rhythm, which continues to work. Sir Elton John received a pacemaker in 1999. Sir Roger Moore, the 007 actor, received a pacemaker after blacking out on stage in 2003. An overactive thyroid gland (hyperthyroidism) was reportedly the cause of the former president George H.W. Bush's atrial fibrillation episode in 1991. Former Vice President Dick Cheney missed campaign events in 2008 because of AF and his heart rhythm was restored with cardio version—a short electrical shock to the heart. The most common treatment today is a same-day radiofrequency ablation or cryosurgery (freezing) of the heart's short-circuiting malfunction, to restore normal rhythm. Close to 1 million people per year are being so treated in the United Kingdom, thus reducing the incidence of crippling or fatal strokes.

Dr Emanuel argued the United States should stop focusing on extending life as the chief priority, and instead focus on quality of life. He said claims of "morbidity compression," the belief that in living longer, people will be healthier longer, simply isn't proving to be true. Instead, people are now living sicker longer. (This concern is covered later). It would seem, however, that Dr Emanuel is wrong about the failure of compression of morbidity, as the latest Harvard study (June

2016) found that the increase in life expectancy in the past two decades has been accompanied by an even greater increase in life years free of disability.[25]

For the typical person, once you reach age 65, you can likely look forward to years of healthy activity and disability-free life. The Harvard study found that in 1992, the life expectancy of the average 65-year-old was 17.5 years, 8.9 of which were free from disability. By 2008, total life expectancy had risen to 18.8 years. In addition to the overall increase, the number of disability-free years increased, from 8.9 to 10.7, while the number of disabled years fell, from 8.6 to 8.1.

Driving those changes are two major treatment areas—cardiovascular health and vision treatment. There has been an incredibly dramatic decline in deaths and disabilities from heart disease and heart failure. Some of it is the result of people smoking less, and better diet, but it is estimated that as much as half of the improvement is because of medical care, especially statin drug treatment, which is both preventing heart attacks and improving people's recovery. Much of the improvement in vision health can be summed up in a single word—cataracts. In the past, cataract surgery was very lengthy and technically difficult, whereas that same surgery today can be done in an outpatient setting, so that complications and disability are significantly ameliorated. While improved treatment for heart disease and vision problems have significantly added to disability-free life expectancy, some conditions—particularly dementia, neuro-degenerative disorders like Parkinson's disease and chronic-disabling conditions like diabetes—remain a concern."[26]

This is great news, as these reported years of disability have fallen significantly since I started researching this book. There is even more we can do, to Live even Longer and Better without disabilities and with minimal drugs.

I do, however, agree with Dr Emanuel and Shannon Brownlee, senior vice president of the Lown Institute (which I presume is named after Nobel Prize winner Bernard Lown, MD, inventor of the defibrillator and introducer of lidocaine into medical practice), in their efforts to reform healthcare for the aging: "The pressure to undergo more tests, more treatments, and more invasive procedures as one gets older and frailer comes from all sides—from friends, from the hospital, from well-meaning clinicians... We need to make it easier for people to resist futile or unwanted treatments—to say no."[27] It is hard to disagree with Emanuel and Brownlee that interfering, intrusive and invasive tests should not be done when old patients are ill and there is no real hope of improving their quality of life. Here I couldn't agree more with them.

And if struck down with some serious or terminal illness consigning us to a nursing home with the aforementioned indignities, then, I agree, Dr Emanuel may well have a point. In fact, just this week I examined a vivacious young lawyer who worked for a large law firm and whose job was litigating aged care. She was a very pretty girl but her face clouded over when discussing this subject. She vehemently advised me a number of times to "never go into a nursing home" and sketched out for me just the superficial horrors she saw as a lawyer; let alone the medical horrors. She appeared so affected by her experience that I doubt very much if she will, or can, continue in this branch of the law. And if I were an oncologist (cancer specialist) or a nursing home doctor I think I too would like to bow out at 75 rather than endure the seemingly unavoidable progressive indignities and degradation.

Perhaps, however, a finite 75-year lifespan does not fit all. Given the right information, there are now ways to predict and therefore avoid those most critical illnesses and live (and work) much longer. There is also evidence indicating how to stay healthier; not smoking is the best known, but there are now many other evidenced lifestyles, which are not onerous nor will make us into health freaks. And while Dr Emanuel states he doesn't want any interventions, there are many advances in modern medicine, such as cataract surgery, artificial hips and radiofrequency heart ablation, that return a near blind, hobbling invalid or a potential stroke victim to being effectively normal rather than languishing and deteriorating, waiting for a premature and avoidable death.

10. Living Well Past 75

I simply contend that living past 75 is possible for most of us. In fact recent medical advances now confirm this with documented evidence and methods. Sir Richard Doll, at 92, and my father who practiced medicine until he was 84, have demonstrated that it is possible to live longer, past 75, remaining healthy, happy and productive with only a final short, dignified, fatal illness at an old age. There is now evidence for how to avoid or cure previous, seemingly inevitable illnesses without much expense or restrictions.

When Dr Emanuel expressed his death wish at 75 years of age, the Queen was 90, Prince Phillip 93, President Carter and Bush Sr 90; and even though Jimmy Carter now has liver cancer and melanoma, he has lived more than 15 years beyond 75. Meanwhile, Catherine Hamlin, a medical colleague, was 91 and still working in Ethiopia while the newspaper proprietor, Rupert Murdoch, was 84 and I see "just married"; satirist and comedian Barrie Humphries was still filling theatres at 81; and Buzz Aldrin, the second man on the Moon (whose mother's maiden name was "Moon") was still touring the world urging funding for the space trip to Mars. Then also alive were Sean Connery, of James Bond fame, at 84; and Dirty Harry, Clint Eastwood; while SeeSee Rigney, an Operating Room Nurse at Tacoma General Hospital, was still working and celebrated her 90th birthday on 7 May 2015. President Obama interviewed David Attenborough, the BBC Naturalist, on his 89th birthday in May 2015, and it was a lucid and delightful interview. In October 2014 the following were also steaming along in their 75th year or older: Raquel Welch, Martin Sheen, Jane Fonda, Judi Dench, Tina Turner, Patrick Stewart, Faye Dunaway, Diahann Carroll, Nick Nolte, Al Pacino, Dustin Hoffman, Robert Redford and Jack Nicholson, none of whom, to my knowledge, have expressed a desire not to live any longer.

Whetted by this not altogether curious age-75 deadline (literally), I checked, at random to make it superficially statistically valid, the obituaries in *The New York Times* of 10th May 2015, and found that only one person died aged 75! But out of 147 in all, some 110 lived (very well and successfully, according to their obituaries) beyond 75. The most popular age of death, with 12 recorded, was 87, and there were 10 dying at 96 years of age.

In 2016 Denmark's Svend Stensgaard at 93 was the world's oldest licensed power lifter, entering top competitions across the world and lifting up to 150 kg. Even a heart attack 3 years ago hadn't stopped him. In Japan, another 93-year-old, Jun Takahashi, was still flying as the Guinness World Record oldest active commercial pilot. The oldest man to ever climb Mount Everest is Yuichiro Miura who was 80 at the time, while his father skied down Mont Blanc aged 99; and Hidekichi Miyazaki set the record for the over-105-year 100 m race. In 1950 there were 97 centenarians in Japan; in 2015 there were 61,568, of which 54,000 were women. In Britain there were 295 centenarians in 1950 but 14,450 in 2015.

The reason the Japanese live so long is attributed to their traditional diet—rich in fish and lightly cooked vegetables, low in fat and served in modest amounts. Mr Takahashi said, "it's important to stop eating when you are 80% full. I haven't felt completely full for decades and if you want to live a long time, you need to be stylish." This advice conforms to the observations of the "Okinawa Way,"[28] as well as my own observations that pride in one's appearance reflects our internal condition.

The 2014 Public Health Report from England documents that while life expectancy dropped in 2012 and 2013, it recovered in 2014 to be the highest ever recorded, making the maintenance of good health imperative; yet many are living longer in poor health. Women aged 60 should expect to live a further 21 years on average. This means they are now likely to spend a quarter of their life in retirement. At 75 they can expect to live another 13 years, at 85 another 7 years and at 95 another 3 years. Men aged 65 can look forward to another 19 years on average; at 75 another 12 years; at 85, six more years, while at 95 another 3 years. In 2016, Public Health England (PHE) stated that living healthily in midlife can double a person's chances of staying healthy aged 70 and older, with "simple and small" changes. A $7 million media campaign has been allocated, as the NHS spends more than $22 billion a year treating illnesses caused by the effects of bad diet, lack of exercise, smoking and alcohol—with the direct cost of obesity and overweight being estimated at $12 billion a year, lack of exercise $1,800 million a year, and alcohol misuse $7 billion. Forty-two percent of midlife adults are living with at least one long-term health condition, which increases their risk of early death and disability.

When we are young we are bulletproof and make all the mistakes possible (I often state the only reason I'm alive is that the "use by date" on my forehead was smudged) and when we are old we wish we had known how to optimize our lives when we were young. If at an early age we could adopt better eating habits and not indulge in the high-risk behaviors such as smoking and drinking to excess, then 85 and beyond would seem a most realistic objective. It is now stated that 90% of cancers are caused by bad, self-induced practices. Cardiovascular disease (heart attacks and strokes) and cancers are the greatest cause of our dying before 75, but most are preventable; and many previously debilitating illnesses are cured by modern surgery. "Prevention is better than cure"—so if you know what illnesses lie just around the corner, you can adopt an eminently pleasant lifestyle that prevents most illnesses.

The disease-causing properties of smoking were not known until relatively recently, and it used to be high fashion—just watch the old movies—and so people innocently became addicted. The habit certainly shortened their lives, as we now know it causes cancers, cardiovascular disease and more. We are now aware of the dangers and so may not start; armed with this information, a great bulk of the now informed generation don't smoke. But there are many more pieces of information to similarly cut our health risks and ensure we maximize our life span, which don't impose any restrictions or condemn us to a life of onerous deprivation and discipline. An excellent example of this is substituting olive oil for butter, as excellent clinical trials have found it confers benefits. Adding a handful of nuts confers even more benefit. These are not dramatic changes and are easily incorporated and adopted.

11. The New & Previous Evidence

Humans, it has been observed, are at their healthiest when aged 11 years. We are living longer but even so, at present, we can only live the normal human lifespan. While this improvement to longevity will continue, there is now no way to dramatically extend it by much more. The average present population lifespan for most countries peaks at around 80 years. This will continue to extend until the maximum human lifespan is reached. Some feel 120 years of human life may be possible, and a couple of people have indeed reached this age. Living longer, however, comes at a cost, with disabilities and chronic illnesses plaguing our final decades.

The objective of this book is dedicated to *not* dying or being disabled *prematurely*, by optimizing our health to maximize our longevity. Our longevity is, of course, directly linked to our health, and our health is dependent on many interlinked factors.

Factors Affecting Our Health:

Previous Established Criteria

1. Genetics
2. Age
3. Nutrition – the food we eat
4. Weight
5. Hygiene – mainly a clean water supply
6. Environment – where we live – air pollution
7. Medical markers – especially weight, blood pressure, lipids, blood and biochemical profile
8. Exercise
9. Mental status – personality, lack of stress, happiness, Alzheimer's
10. Skin
11. High-risk behaviors

New Criteria (the "Missing Keys")

Health problems and illnesses specific to age and sex

Previous Established Criteria

1. Genetics

We can't alter our genetics but many inherited, genetic or chronic problems such as diabetes 1, coeliac and other autoimmune illnesses can be dramatically ameliorated today with the advances in medicine. Along with such advances, society catches up through education in using, for example, a vastly increased range of tasty gluten-free foods.

2. Age

Age is the greatest risk factor for our health.

Atrial fibrillation, where the heart beats rapidly, is now an age-related epidemic, along with osteoarthritis, reduced eyesight, and poorer dentition. While these conditions may be obvious, less obvious ones such as reduced hearing can be part of increased social isolation which contributes to premature demise.

One of the great tragedies I encounter almost daily are patients who simply have never addressed these inevitable age changes and are simply bewildered and devastated when illness strikes or their spouse dies. To live past 75 you should plan your old age now—and not just you. Think what your spouse will do if you depart. The key to this, after coping with the grief, is social integration and mobilization—friends, clubs, hobbies are absolutely essential. If you are under 50 this may seem all too far away. It is tragic when those in their 70s and older just won't face it and plan accordingly; then the survivor often becomes a recluse with an ever accelerating downward spiral as to their own personal care and health.

3. Nutrition – or as I choose to call it, "Newtrition" – the food we eat

A Global Survey concluded that "Poor diet is consistently responsible for more disease and death than physical inactivity, smoking and alcohol combined".[4]

See "Newtrition" Book 2 for much greater detail. One studied type of diet

---

[4]Global Burden of Diseases, Injuries, and Risk Factors Study 2013. *The Lancet*, 22 Jul 2014.

led to a 56% *increase* in cardiovascular disease, while another reduced heart attacks by 76%. Which food plan do you want?

Recently I examined a not overweight gas station attendant who, like most of us today, is working longer harder and feels “too tired” to cook when he gets home at night. Instead he feeds up on the processed food at his Servo—sausage rolls, with their high saturated fat pastry and dubious contents, were his nominated favorite. He may not be overweight now but our modern lifestyle and access to prepared processed, cheap and delicious food does not augur well for his future. When I ran through my Newtrition advice he agreed it was good and he liked it... but would never do it. The processed food was simply too easy and convenient. At least he was a realist and not blaming anyone else.

You will have to make an effort, which is why this book is for the motivated individual. The government is not going to home-deliver healthy food to you, do your exercise or organize the other proven preventive health measures.

4. Weight

See Fast Start Pages Précis at end or Book 4 for the complete plan.

Losing weight is the hardest thing we can do in an affluent society with delicious junk food, researched to make you want more, advertised and available in excess 24 hours a day, seven days a week and home-delivered. Most, in fact all, fad diets don’t work long-term, but I provide the evidence as to the actual researched best way to lose fat.

The 'Obesity Paradox' is a fable: for each 5-unit increase in BMI above 25 kg/m2, the corresponding increases in risk were 49% for cardiovascular mortality, 38% for respiratory disease mortality, and 19% for cancer mortality. The hazards of excess body weight were greater in younger than in older people and in men than in women.[29]

5. Hygiene

Hygiene is mainly the province of public health / government authorities and requires a clean water supply and a good sewerage system. Recent epidemics such as Ebola and bird flu demonstrate the need for personal improvements. The introduction of antibiotics has made us all blasé. We now feel disdain for illnesses which struck terror into the population prior to the introduction of antibiotics in the mid-1930s; so now we don’t wash our hands (even doctors) and we cough and sneeze over all and sundry, thus spreading flu and respiratory infections. There are, however, many everyday behaviors which can better protect us and these are covered in a later Book.

6. Environment – where we live

Western societies with 24-hour availability of junk food have seen the development of the "Diseases of Affluence": *Heart Disease, Strokes, Hypertension, Hyperlipidemia* and *Obesity*, with the resulting downstream conditions *Diabetes 2, Depression* and *Arthritis*. The Sun Belt (across the southern United States) is witnessing an epidemic of melanoma and skin cancers. Polluted air is linked to 1.6 million deaths a year in China;[30] and no matter where we live there are some 80,000 untested chemicals, invented since WW2, in our water and food containers. The sperm counts of Swedish fishermen have dropped (it is alleged from the dioxin from timber mills spilling into the sea and being eaten by the fish) while similar pollution of the water has witnessed English freshwater fish and Florida alligators becoming hermaphroditic.

The increasing world population is already polluting previously clean if not pristine areas including rain forests. While humans are gregarious animals and seem drawn to big cities, the famous experiment where enforced overcrowding of rats saw them lose their hair and become more aggressive would seem to suggest there is a limit. Even the imposition and intrusion of new technology such as wind-farms into a previously untouched area might have yet-to-be-determined long-term effects. Drones, mobile phone cameras, the official or undetected collecting of personal information by hacking or legitimate commercial means as in "Predictive Analysis," all would now seem to make privacy a thing of the past. Such intrusions and increased expectations and work pressures provoke obvious and not obvious stress, the outcome of which is becoming more and more apparent.

Air pollution has now been found to cause up to 30% of strokes. The pollution from car fumes, especially diesel, in cities is well known. Sitting in traffic immediately behind the car in front's exhaust is the worst—so close all vents. A screen of trees can prevent the exhaust from intruding into our homes.

7. Medical markers

Weight, blood pressure, blood glucose, lipids, blood and biochemical profile are fundamental. Hand in hand with these are the newer investigations and tests that can better identify conditions early so preventive measures can be instituted. One example is coronary artery calcium screening. I was an early advocate of this and watched as the medical journals endlessly debated its worth—which of course should be done. In the end, it was found useful and is now widely used as a screening test. My enthusiasm arose when I was screening an eye surgeon whose every other parameter, including both his Routine and Stress ECG/EKG, were normal, but he had chest pains; and, while it was not yet an approved test, we found his coronary calcium was very high. He nearly retired then and there. That was 2002. He is still operating today, 15 years later.

8. Exercise

See Book 4 for the complete plan. Overall, while exercise doesn't bring about much weight loss, it is still the best value health investment for the money. Cycling to work has been found to reduce all cause mortality and deaths from cerebrovascular disease and cancers. Walking was not as good.

9. Mental status

For normal emotions, albeit extreme, such as the grief of the death of one's partner, which we once coped with by emotional support and time, we now expect some pill to alleviate or even cure. Our vulnerability is exploited by ruthless Big Pharma (drug companies) such that "depression" is considered an epidemic, and their profits at record levels. In 2008 the NEJM published an article that reviewed over 70 major studies of antidepressants. Thirty-eight showed positive results, and most of these were published. Of the remaining 36 showing negative results, 22 were buried, and 11 were published giving a positive slant; only three were published accurately.[31]

It is no longer bad parenting or drugs while pregnant which causes ADD (Attention Deficit Disorder), for which "more drugs are needed" even though recently they have been shown to be of little worth.

While there is no doubt that these psychiatric disorders exist, what I am suggesting is that drug therapy is not always needed. A review of one's lifestyle and coping strategies, and cognitive behavioral therapy may be the first priority. Dementia and Alzheimer's is covered in Book 3.

10. Skin

Living in the Sun Belt, or increased holidays when we bake in the sun, don't wear sunglasses or cover up, have resulted in an epidemic of skin cancer and melanoma. However, some daily sun exposure is important for health. Nonsmokers who stayed out of the sun had a life expectancy similar to smokers who soaked up the most rays, according to researchers who studied nearly 30,000 Swedish women over 20 years. This finding indicates that avoiding the sun "is a risk factor for death of a similar magnitude as smoking." Women who seek out the sun were generally at lower risk for cardiovascular disease (CVD) and noncancerous/non-CVD diseases such as diabetes, multiple sclerosis, and pulmonary diseases, than those who avoided sun exposure. An increased risk of skin cancer was found in the study, but the skin cancers that occurred in those exposing themselves had a better prognosis.[32]

The worst behavior is fair-skinned people "binge-burning"—getting severe exposure and burning rather than acquiring a gradual tan. The above study was done in Sweden where the sun is not so intense and sun cancer rates are low in any event; whereas Queensland, closer to the equator, has the highest incidence of skin cancer in the world. While some sun exposure would seem a good thing, the duration should lessen when closer to the equator.

11. High-Risk Behaviors

High-risk behaviors are lifestyle actions that increase medical problems. These are not obviously dangerous escapades such as base jumping or mountaineering, but everyday habits, which account for over 50% of health problems. See Chapter 1:

Then there are other pursuits wherein we accept the risks but without really realizing how dangerous these risks are: A prospective study of 40 retired National Football League players finds that over 40% show MRI evidence of traumatic brain injury. Participants (average age, 36) showed "significant abnormalities in attention and concentration (42%), executive function (50%), [and] learning/memory (44.7%)."[34] While NFL and boxing head injuries should be obvious and can cause Parkinson's disease, we underestimate the risks in many other sports, which do not appear as violent. However, heading the ball in soccer, especially when wet, has also been documented as causing long-term brain injury.

With the death of Mohammed Ali, the devastating effects of Parkinson's disease on this formerly magnificent athlete were there for all to see. There is no definite proof that the repeated head trauma was the cause, but it has to be the number-one suspect. By coincidence a classmate who was the school boxing champion also died, at the same age, on the same day, from Parkinson's disease. Head trauma can be the cause of Parkinson's disease, and participants of all violent sports, such as boxing and football, with their repeated head blows, and soccer with the repeated heading of the ball, must be aware of the danger.

And Not Just Youths

Skateboard accidents cause around 180 hospital visits a day in the United States. Squash balls and champagne corks cause many eye injuries. Quad bikes, then tractors, are the greatest cause of farm deaths and serious injuries. Angle grinders are the most dangerous of tradesmen-handyman tools.

I am not advocating that we cocoon ourselves in cotton wool, but I am advocating that we are fully made aware of the dangers so we can minimize the risks. How tragic it is to read how kids were killed on a quad bike because they perceived it as a fun vehicle and no one told them otherwise, gave them a helmet or a seatbelt.

Had I known such risks would I have changed my habits? You bet! I played (too) many years of rugby when hard knocks were never admitted to but I gave up my skateboard (in my 50s) when I read how a champion athlete my age had fallen off his and broken his hip. My friend's squash racquet opened my eyebrow but my eye at least remained intact. I now know how to hold in and control a champagne cork after I witnessed one actually hitting someone in the eye. When the angle grinder kicked back I couldn't believe how sudden, violet and dangerous it was; and having owned three quad bikes, I only wish the man who sold us the first one had warned us of the inherent design dangers (they tip over very easily if turned too sharply). No one over 60 should climb a ladder, let alone stand on a chair to reach or fix something. My mother rang me to say my 86-year-old father "couldn't get up." He had been standing on a chair putting up kitchen curtains and wouldn't believe my "spot diagnosis" of a fractured neck of his femur (thigh bone). The injured person lies in a characteristic position so the diagnosis can be made immediately. Like most formerly active men he didn't know when not to pursue activities which may not have been dangerous when younger. One surgeon I knew slipped off his ladder cleaning out the gutters of his roof and ended up being a vegetable in a nursing home. Do I get up on chairs to get the special condiments? Well, yes, but I am very aware of the risks and make sure it is a solid wooden chair and that I have supports. My excuse is that I do know the dangers, unlike most men, and I am super careful. This gets back to not wrapping ourselves in cotton wool: we can continue most of our previous activities if we know the dangers and how to avoid them.

New Criteria – Evidence: Specific Problems Related to Age and Sex

The new evidence as set out in the tables in the next two chapters lists, in order, the causes of deaths, then disabilities. Later chapters list the prevalence of illnesses and why we visit our doctor. These are incredibly revealing, as they allow focus on the key risk factors for the illnesses we should concentrate on, for each decade and sex. They also reveal little-known facts that most young people don't think about until it's too late—such as hearing impairment, which is often preventable but condemns the person to a great deal of social isolation in their old age. The rock concerts, the boom boxes, the surround high-volume car speakers, the earphones, all are harbingers of deafness; and deafness is one of the worst causes of social isolation and loneliness. But do my warnings fall on deaf ears already? Just today I examined a 73-year-old, very alert and good-looking Dutch woman who had just paid $6,000 for her hearing aids that didn't work very well and, delightful as she was, she agonized over how she was becoming progressively isolated, as she was too embarrassed to keep asking people to repeat themselves. Yesterday I diagnosed a hideous cancer on the leg of a 70-year-old who complained that no one advised him to cover up or use sunscreen to go surfing, with its dangers of sun exposure, when he was younger.

Screening

A recent study concluded that screening is overused for some diseases and that it is possibly perceived as more effective and cost-effective than it is. However, the study does advise that "the role of screening should be considered on a disease-specific basis,"[35] which is exactly what this book does.

Many illnesses are not preventable, but most are, or are eminently treatable if diagnosed early. But we must be aware of what they are and when they are most likely to "attack" us. If we have this information, if we know when and where the enemy is, we are at least and at last in a position to fight back. Yet every day we blunder in making dangerous medical mistakes, which accumulate to shorten our lives or to cause us to become housebound, or nursing home invalids.[36]

Cost-Effective Prevention

An initial basic approach to preventive measures, as below, costs no more and in fact should save money. The aim is either not to start, or to stop, those habits or behaviors which are proven to shorten life or cause illness. While smoking is incredibly expensive and deleterious, so is excessive booze. Meanwhile one of the hidden costs, the expenses "that dare not be mentioned," are for vitamins, supplements, so-called health foods and gimmicks. These are invariably not needed, so the cost savings can be significant; but the true believers who swallow them seem to be in denial as to those costs.

Some observers point to the medical costs of living longer: "There's also the unavoidable fact that every time you prevent people from dying from one disease, they are likely to live longer and incur future medical expenses. The patient who benefits from cholesterol screening may go on to develop cancer, arthritis, Alzheimer's or some other costly illnesses."[37] I would contend this view is simplistic.

Do you not test for diabetes, a very costly illness, and just let them die? Or do you do a blood glucose test which costs a couple of dollars, or even a urine dip-stick which costs a couple of cents, and identify patients who, if they just change their diet, can live healthier and longer, working and paying taxes?

Live Longest is all about cost-effective prevention. It is pointed out in Newtrition, in Book 2, that "bad nutrition is now the greatest health problem of the Western world"; and while fresh produce may cost more, it is cost-effective because of its health benefits.

Basic Cost-Effective Measures:

Adopting ***the Newtrition PHYTO Diet (Book 2)*** means there is no need for vitamins or supplements plus profound health benefits.

Daily exercise / activity / not sedentary—no gym necessary

BMI < 27 (normal weight)

No smoking

Moderate drinking

Normal Blood Pressure (BP)

Normal Low-Density cholesterol (LDL)

Normal Blood Glucose (BG)

Vaccinations

Be happy, acceptance, meditation

The first five cost no more and, in fact, save money and may lead to normal BP, LDL and BG. The cost savings for both individuals and the Nation would be incredible, with the compression of morbidity–living healthier longer. But politicians are scared to legislate or discriminate *against* the obese or the sick, however, giving tax deductions for achieving each of the above targets would surely encourage a healthier lifestyle on a national scale.

Higher diet quality scores have been consistently associated with a lower risk of mortality. All-cause mortality was reportedly reduced by 11–42%, cardiovascular disease mortality by 17–60% and cancer mortality by 11–40% in individuals with the highest category of scores of diet quality compared with individuals with the lowest category.[38] Fresh fruit and vegetables may initially cost more than processed junk, but as you can see, not in the long term.

At this stage I must inject a plea. Yesterday I examined a fit-looking man in his 50s who had an eminently treatable heart condition, as did my piano player. Both, however, had their priorities wrong. My piano player spent his money elsewhere (mostly on women) and wouldn't pay to get his heart fixed and died suddenly. This business consultant also didn't want to pay to get his heart fixed but told me he was flying to Auckland to see his old Rugby team play and "would drop [spend] $2000," something he apparently did regularly. There does seem a body of people who are reluctant to spend money on their health, especially if there are free or subsidized health schemes available, which both of these men had access to and were waiting for. If you are dead or an invalid, all the sex or rugby in the world is of no use to you. Get your priorities right: Health is Number 1. Spend money there first—from fruit to heart procedures.

"Life's a bitch, then you die": so goes the old cynical saying, and just telling someone to "be happy" doesn't do it. You have to work at it. Finding what you like, not taking on too much while challenging yourself, and reducing stress are a start, but meditation has also been found to work. Later books cover Happiness, Stress and Meditation.

While we are living longer than our forbears, this has been mainly due to public health measures: better hospitals and births, cleaner water and sewerage, more hygienic food preparation, vaccinations and the eradication or minimization of previous scourges (measles, polio, typhoid, TB, to name a few). Antibiotics have not made much of a dint in terms of overall improvement to the health of the population, except each of us individually must surely be thankful for their miracle. All of this progress, however, does not contradict the ***Live Longest*** avowed aim to optimize our personal health and maximize our longevity. These public health measures raised the living standards and health for the population as a whole, but the specialized fine-tuning and changes now provided and recommended are beyond the funds or legislation of any government. These are initiatives and improvements you do yourself, which is why Americans, as individuals, live longer.

Medications

As a physician I fully realize some medications are necessary. My attitude is to minimize them in general and also to use the minimum effective dose. The tragic truth, however, is that it is easier to take a pill than run (or even walk) around the block, so the bulk (pun intended) of us prefer to take pills. It is no use "ordering" patients to take preventive measures, but as reported in the *BMJ* in 2015, "Falls in blood pressure and total cholesterol staved off more than 20,000 deaths from coronary heart disease in England between 2000 and 2007." Only a small proportion (1800) of the blood pressure segment (numbering 13,000) were attributable to drug treatment, with the rest accounted for by changes in risk factors at the population level. Falls in total cholesterol accounted for some 7400 deaths prevented or postponed, of which 5300 were attributable to statins, with the remainder attributable to changes in risk factors at the population level. It was concluded that population-wide approaches focusing on prevention, such as public health initiatives to curb salt and trans fat levels in processed and take-away foods, may have more of an impact than prescribing drugs to individuals.[39] To this we may well add reduction in processed foods and sugar.

Overall

Knowing what illnesses can strike us, and when, is such an obvious preventive health strategy that I am staggered that, until now, it has not become standard recommended practice. Perhaps these statistics are so relatively new that the information hasn't trickled down. Preventive medicine is not really practiced or practiced as best it can, using all the now available information.

There is, of course, a big overlap between death and disability (see next chapters). If a heart attack doesn't kill you it can leave you a cardiac cripple. You may survive a stroke intellectually intact but be paralyzed down one side. The colon cancer may have been excised but the colostomy bag compromises your former work and social activities. The road accident left you with brain damage... and so on. These are disabilities caused by what otherwise would have caused death.

We all have to die of something... but later, not sooner! What this book is all about is preventing or avoiding illnesses and conditions that can kill or disable us sooner than our natural lifespan allows. They can overlap or can be widely different, but knowing what can occur, and when, can help us avoid them.

In the mid-1990s a great leap forward in medical records and statistics was instituted. Decade-by-decade statistics now allow information as to the

Causes of Premature Deaths (next chapter)
Causes of Non-Fatal Burdens of Disease (NFBD) (next chapter after the above)
Most Prevalent Health Conditions (later following chapters)
Most Common Reason For Attending a Doctor (later following chapters)

In a later chapter the statistics show the incredible sudden, usually unrecognized, deteriorations at age 40:

Cardiovascular Disease
Blood pressure
Cholesterol
Diabetes
Cancer
Lung Disease
Rheumatoid Arthritis
Osteoporosis and Osteoarthritis
Eyesight
Weight

All of the above get "suddenly" worse at around age 40. But this onslaught is not really sudden. It is not the first puff of a cigarette that causes the lung cancer or the one sunburn that causes the melanoma, but rather the repeated exposure to these irritant carcinogens. In the same way, it is not the one bad meal that causes the cardiovascular disease, hyperlipidemia, overweight and diabetes, but rather the long-term, chronic abuse of our bodies by high-risk habits and behaviors from that peak-health age of 11 (if not before, even in the womb). Like lung cancer or a melanoma which may seem "sudden," they all are, in fact, just the end result of long-term abuse. The good news, however, is that it's never too late to reverse or improve much of this damage.

By combining all the tables, which follow, it is now possible to provide the most complete picture of our health possible. Not all countries have such in-depth statistics, but for Western countries these figures provide a similar basis. By combining the lists of Causes of Death with those of Illness Burden, a more complete picture of our health emerges.

Go to your country (USA/UK/Australia), find your age group and sex, and find what illnesses are most likely to affect you. These are the ones you should screen for. More extensive lists are to be found with each country's health authorities: USA = Center for Disease Control (CDC); UK = National Statistics; Australia = Australian Institute of Health and Welfare (AIHW).

National, Ethnic and Social Differences

There are significant national differences. While high-risk behavior in young males is universal, the United States adds a greater dimension to this, with homicide featuring for both sexes up to 35, and beyond for men.

There are also socioeconomic class differences. I stand to be corrected but I would think homicide is more prevalent in deprived areas than the affluent or educated suburbs.

The figures for suicide are alarming and probably shadow depression, which is not an official cause of death.

I cannot explain the high rates of poisoning. Maybe it's related to suicide.

"Liver Disease" covers a multitude of illnesses from hepatitis to cirrhosis, with hepatitis C and cirrhosis often being self-inflicted by drug use and alcohol.

Concurrent Illnesses

Overall the disease that kills most of us as we age is coronary heart disease (CAD), but what is not listed is that it often accompanied by hypertension (HT), obesity, hyperlipidemia (cholesterol) and diabetes.

Lung cancer and lung diseases, which also feature prominently, are usually the result of smoking, which, again, is preventable.

Changes Over Time

Some statistics have altered slightly since I first researched them. The order or incidence of these illnesses have altered slightly from 1996 (published 2000) to 2003 (published 2004) and on until the latest iteration. This is to be expected as prevention has improved. For example, decreased male smoking has seen lung cancer drop from second to third.

The overwhelming fact remains that cardiovascular disease remains the leading cause of death and burden for both sexes. If it doesn't kill you prematurely, it will turn you into a dependent invalid more so than any other illness.

Prescribed Drugs

One statistic has been understandably, but disturbingly, missing. That is the problems caused by prescribed drugs or medical errors. It was listed here at number six in the combined list, but some authorities have felt it may be as high as fourth; and now medical errors have been alleged as being the third leading cause of hospital death;[40] but there is room for doubt, as noted elsewhere.

In an article titled "My Top Six Easily Preventable Causes of Patient Death and Morbidity," Dr Melissa Wilson-Shirley listed her third as "Discharging the Patient on All the Same Drugs That Weren't Working When They Were Admitted,"[41] which conforms to my experience as mentioned below.

More Elderly Using Dangerous Drug Combinations

One in six older adults now regularly use potentially deadly combinations of prescription and over-the-counter medications and dietary supplements—a twofold increase over a 5-year period. While it is not known how many older adults in the United States die of drug interactions, the risk seems to be growing, and public awareness is lacking.[42]

If you are taking any medications, see what can be reduced or stopped. Recently it has been found that:

- Many statins are now not needed, as the heart risk calculators were wrong. But they are beneficial if needed.
- Aspirin is not recommended for primary cardiovascular prevention.
- NSAIDS cause bleeding and heart attacks.
- PPIs for heartburn increase the risk of heart attacks and dementia.

As a young Medical Registrar my first action on admitting a patient was to "cease all medications." At the time of admission I well remember many patients taking over 15 different drugs; and one (which I think represents a personal record) was on some 33 different drugs. Most of these patients when later discharged, feeling much better, were only taking the three or four essential drugs actually needed.

Obviously the doctor is not trying to poison his patient and, too often, the patient is reluctant to complain of side effects. Frequently, when seeing different doctors a new drug is added but an old one is not ceased. However, all drugs have side effects, so it behooves the patient *to balance their greater benefit against any downside*. Many people have idiosyncratic responses to even the most common drugs. So don't ignore side effects; note any new problems that occur after you start any new medication; and *get your whole medication regime reviewed at least annually*. Make a specific appointment just for this and nothing else.

And, when all else fails, read the instructions. Most drugs "fail" because patients don't take them correctly, if at all. It has been found that many patients are too polite to refuse the doctor's prescription and never get it filled. Why, then, do they go to the doctor?

Older patients are being prescribed numerous "invisible" anticholinergic drugs that put them at risk of side effects such as cognitive impairment. While drugs for urinary incontinence and tricyclic antidepressants are traditionally recognised for their high-level anticholinergic risks, most of the anticholinergic burden for elderly patients comes from the unwitting prescribing of low-level anticholinergic drugs.

The top 8 anticholinergic drugs to be beware of:[43]

1. Warfarin
2. Oxycodone
3. Frusemide
4. Prednisolone
5. Prochlorperazine
6. Digoxin
7. Fentanyl
8. Morphine

But Worse

It has been reported that there is an out-of-control epidemic in the United States that costs more and affects more people than any disease Americans currently worry about. It is reasonable to conclude that this is also the case in other first world countries.

It's called nonadherence to prescribed medications, and it is potentially 100% preventable by the very individuals it afflicts.

The numbers are staggering. According to a review in Annals of Internal Medicine[5] "Studies have consistently shown that 20% to 30% of medication prescriptions are never filled, and that approximately 50% of medications for chronic disease are not taken as prescribed." People who do take prescription medications – whether it's for a simple infection or a life-threatening condition – typically take only about half the prescribed doses. This lack of adherence, the Annals observed, is estimated to cause approximately 125,000 deaths and at least 10% of hospitalizations, and to cost the American health care system between $100 billion and $289 billion a year.

2016: Work Schedule Is Top Barrier to Staying Healthy[44]

The Mayo Clinic National Health Check-Up studies Americans' health opinions and behaviors, from barriers to getting healthy to perceptions of aging. Work schedule was considered as the top barrier to health.

Top Health Resolutions for 2016

1. Eat a healthier diet (74%)
2. Exercise more (73%)
3. Schedule an annual wellness visit with your doctor (66%).

Women were more likely than men to say that they will do something to improve their health in 2016:

---

[5] Interventions to improve adherence to self-administered medications for chronic diseases in the United States: a systematic review. Ann Intern Med. 2012 Dec 4;157(11):785-95.

- Eat a healthier diet (80% vs. 67%)
- Schedule an annual wellness visit with their doctor (70% vs. 62%)
- Get more sleep (67% vs. 58%)
- See their doctor to discuss symptoms they have been experiencing (62% vs. 51%)
- Take a nutritional supplement (63% vs. 47%)
- Schedule a milestone screening (56% vs. 26%)

It was concerning that fewer men planned to schedule a milestone screening, such as a colonoscopy, in 2016. It was recommended that men need to prioritize screenings. If they are of average risk, men should begin getting screened for colorectal and prostate cancer at age 50, and sooner if they are of above-average risk.

Inflammation

Inflammation occurs naturally in the body; but chronic inflammation, which we may not notice, is now considered as often initiating many other illnesses, and therefore it may provide an early warning system to prevent them. Some of these disorders involve the immune system as well as many major diseases, including cancer, heart disease (atherosclerosis was previously considered a bland lipid storage disease), diabetes and Alzheimer's disease. It is thought that statins may reduce heart disease by reducing this inflammation.

Chronic inflammation has been shown to create successions of destructive reactions that damage cells, thus playing a major role in the development of age-related diseases such as cancer, heart disease, and dementia. According to the Centers for Disease Control and Prevention (CDC), seven of the top 10 causes of death in 2010 were chronic diseases, with heart disease and cancer accounting for nearly 48% of all deaths. The CDC also reports in that same year 86% of all health care spending was for people with one or more chronic medical conditions.

Low-grade chronic inflammation is indicated by levels of the inflammatory marker C-reactive protein (CRP).

Some disorders associated with inflammation include:

Acne vulgaris Allergies Asthma Atherosclerosis Autoimmune diseases Autoinflammatory diseases Cancer	Chronic prostatitis Coeliac disease Glomerulonephritis Hypersensitivities Inflammatory bowel diseases Interstitial cystitis Myopathies	Pelvic inflammatory disease Reperfusion injury Rheumatoid arthritis Sarcoidosis Transplant rejection Vasculitis

My simplistic view (as the actual pathological process is a complex cascade of chemicals, enzymes and hormones) is that most inflammation is caused by some irritant. That can include harder-to-digest food; whereas shorter gut transit time with fruit and vegetables is credited with causing less irritation and hence less cancers of the gut. Inflammation is meant to be a protective response, but chronic inflammation can then become an irritant itself. Smoking would seem to be a good example. The smoke contains a number of irritants which bathe the lung cells and then are absorbed into the blood vessels, inflaming all they come into contact with. The lung cells react to this irritant by overgrowing (i.e., cancer). The blood vessels react (inflame) by allowing fat to deposit on the injured surface (i.e., atherosclerosis). Moving on, I feel that processed foods (containing goodness knows what additives and irritants) in prolonged, fermenting contact with the gastrointestinal tract also lead to an inflammatory response and cancer as processed meats seem to do. Non-processed foods, high fiber and rapid transit would seem to just be common sense. Green leafy vegetables also seem to have an endogenous, natural, sulphur-based chemical which may be anti-inflammatory. Aspirin and NSAIDS are also anti-inflammatory and reduce the incidence of colon cancer.

What foods can help fight the risk of chronic inflammation?

Older people are more susceptible to chronic inflammation, so they may benefit from supplementing their diets with isorhamnetin, resveratrol, curcumin and vanillic acid or with food sources that yield these bioactive molecules. Diets rich in fruits and vegetables, which contain polyphenols, protect against age-related inflammation and chronic diseases. Polyphenols are abundant micronutrients in our diet, and evidence for their role in the prevention of degenerative diseases such as cancer and cardiovascular diseases is already emerging.

The health effects of polyphenols depend on the amount consumed and on their bioavailability. Polyphenols derived from onions, turmeric, red grapes, green tea and açai berries may help reduce the release of pro-inflammatory mediators in people at risk of chronic inflammation.[45]

Eating less may help us lead longer, healthier lives. A large, multicenter study reveals that a 25% reduction in calories can significantly lower markers of chronic inflammation without negatively impacting other parts of the immune system.[46]

12. Life Begins At 40?

Physical Declines Begin Earlier Than Expected

New research has confirmed my observations by finding that "physical declines begin sooner in life than typically detected, often when people are still in their 50s. The good news is, with proper attention and effort the ability to function independently can often be preserved with regular exercise. Efforts to maintain basic strength and endurance should begin before age 50, when it's still possible to preserve the skills that keep people mobile and independent later in life." [79] From the following graphs it shows it starts even a decade before this research and we should establish habits of physical effort from 40 years but, as will be seen, even earlier.

These graphs need not be studied in minute detail. What they dramatically show *at a glance* is how most of the pathological changes that prematurely kill or burden us take off at the age of 40. Unfortunately, most of these changes start earlier, go largely unnoticed and only become symptomatic or fatal at a later date.

For those who would prefer to skip the graphs, the conditions covered are:

1. **Cardiovascular disease**
2. **Blood pressure**
3. **Cholesterol**
4. **Diabetes**
5. **Cancer**
6. **Lung disease**
7. **Rheumatoid arthritis**
8. **Osteoporosis and Osteoarthritis**
9. **Eyesight**
10. **Weight**

ALL get worse or rather become symptomatic at around age 40.

A word of caution about these figures:

While these graphs show how these major illnesses dramatically suddenly make their appearance from age 40 they have been asymptomatic but incubating for many years.

We have been "cultivating and incubating" disease conditions certainly since age 11 when we are at the peak of health. It is becoming increasingly likely that the process starts even earlier, with evidence suggesting it may even begin *in utero*. The Vietnam War presented doctors with ostensibly super-fit young men killed in action. Autopsies and post-mortems performed on these young men revealed that many of them, passed as A1 Fit, already had cholesterol/fat deposits in their coronary arteries. While it was not then routine, subsequent autopsies now inspect the coronary arteries of young motor vehicle accident victims, and cholesterol/fat deposits have been found in 11- and even 4-year-old children!

It is common sense that if we continually abuse our bodies, the damage will be cumulative. It's not the one cigarette, it's the small daily dose over 20 or 30 years that causes lung cancer. It's not the one dose of sun but the intermittent or chronic exposure over 40 or more years that results in melanoma. It's not the one fast-food meal but the daily chronic ingestion of bad food that undermines the healthy working of our bodies.

Damage may be in small doses but it is cumulative... so it *"suddenly"* breaks out when we hit 40.

It is never too early to start Preventive Health Lifestyles...nor is it too late.

1. Cardiovascular Disease

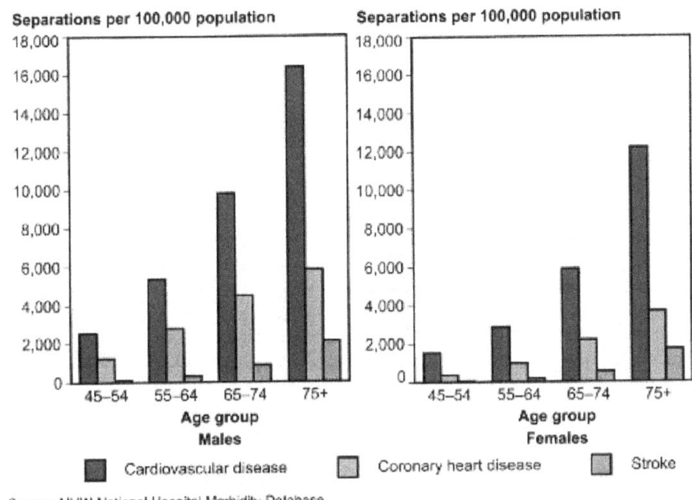

Hospital separations for cardiovascular disease, ages 45 and over

Cardiovascular Disease Takes Off After 40.

2. Blood Pressure

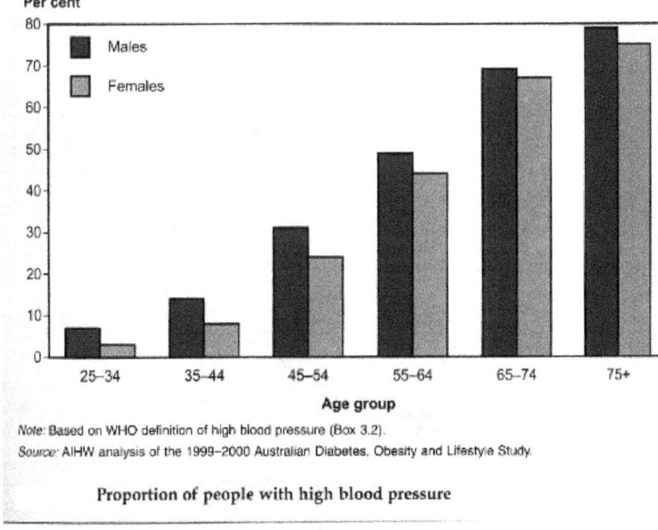

Proportion of people with high blood pressure

Blood Pressure Takes Off After 40.

3. Cholesterol

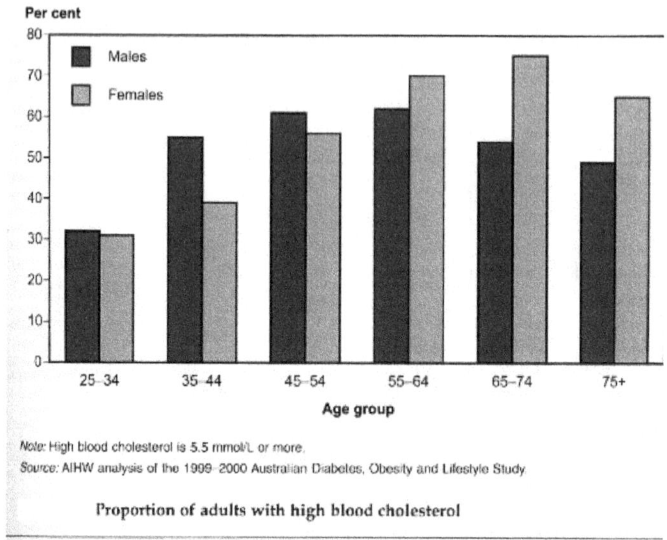

Proportion of adults with high blood cholesterol

Cholesterol Takes Off After 40.

4. Diabetes

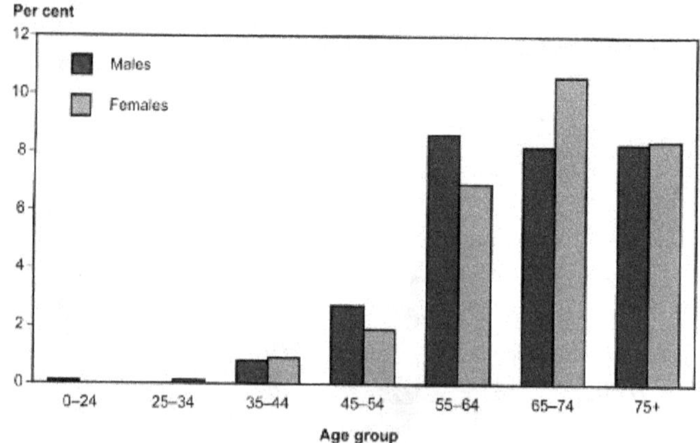

Age-specific prevalence of self-reported Type 2 diabetes

Diabetes Takes Off After 40.

5. Cancer

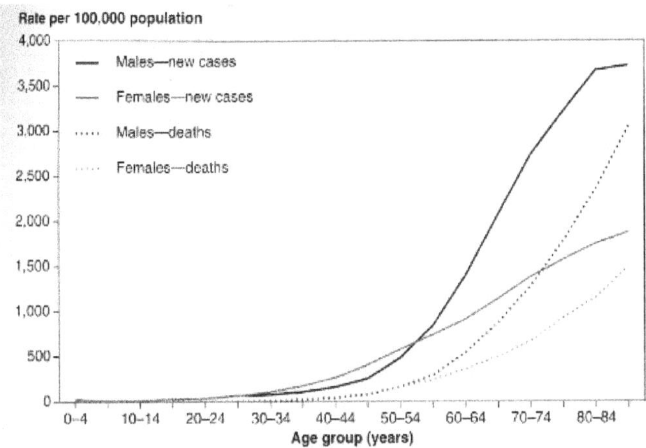

Source: AIHW & AACR 1999.

Age-specific incidence and death rates for malignant neoplasms (excluding non-melanocytic skin cancer), by sex

Cancer Takes Off at 40.

6. Lung Disease

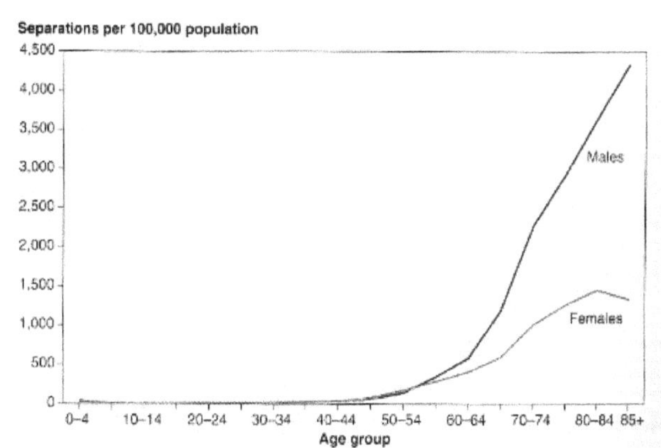

Source: AIHW National Hospital Morbidity Database.

Age-specific hospital separations with COPD as the principal diagnosis

Lung Disease Takes Off at 40.

7. Rheumatoid arthritis

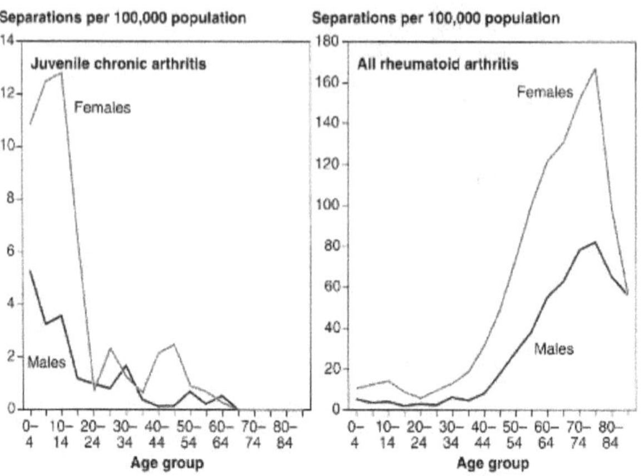

Age-specific hospital separations with principal diagnoses of juvenile chronic arthritis and rheumatoid arthritis

Rheumatoid Arthritis Takes Off at 40.

8. Osteoporosis and Osteoarthritis

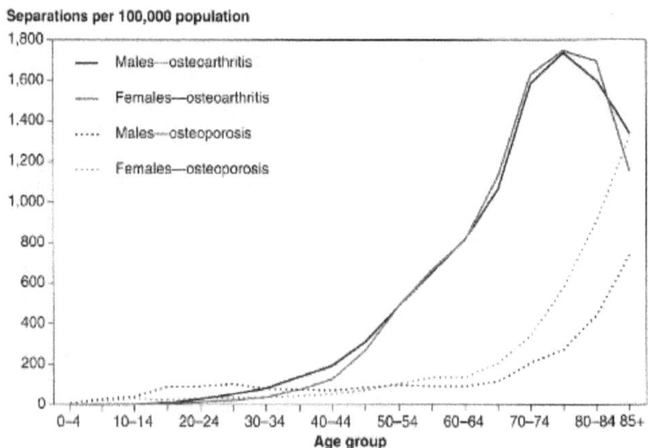

Age-specific hospital separations with principal diagnoses of osteoporosis and osteoarthritis

Osteoarthritis and Osteoporosis Take Off at 40.

9. Eyesight

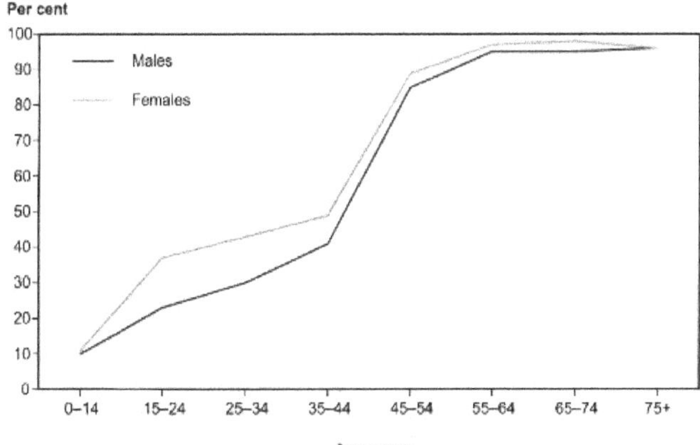

Self-reported prevalence of sight problems

Eyesight Deteriorates at 40.

10. Weight

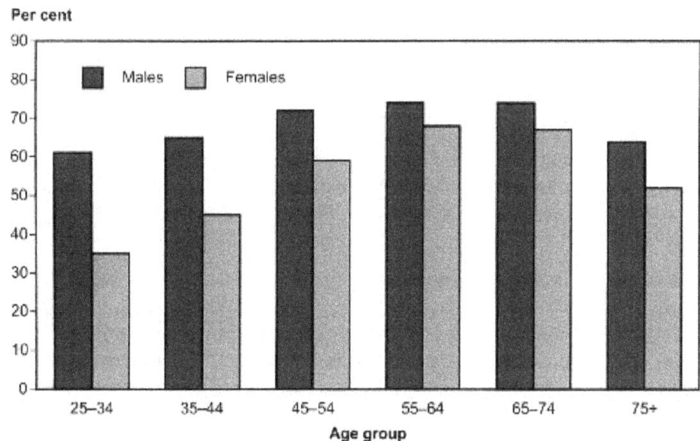

Proportion of people who are overweight (BMI of 25 or more)

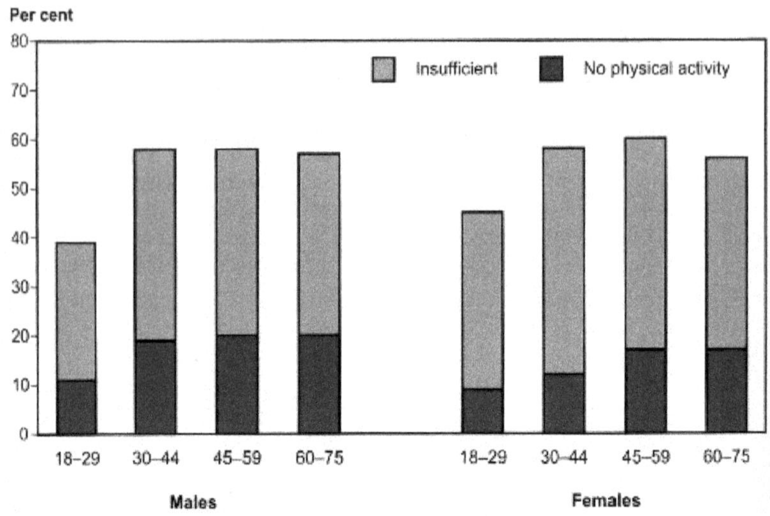

Notes

1. Age-standardised to the 2001 Australian population.
2. People aged 18–75 years.
3. 'Insufficient physical activity' is less than 150 minutes or less than five sessions of physical activity in the previous week.

Source: AIHW analysis of the 2000 National Physical Activity Survey.

Proportion of adults undertaking insufficient or no physical activity

The weight graph above shows that even young people, aged 25 to 34 years (60% of males and 35% of females) are overweight. This is a significant finding, and perhaps the most revealing of all the graphs, as it is the only one where we can actually see that unhealthy practices are cumulative and gradually lead to a health problem, which seemingly takes off after 40. Most of the other illnesses, which take off after 40, show no signs or symptoms even though they have been `brewing" for years. Weight gain, however, is visible at any age, even if we don't see it for ourselves. The second graph shows the amount of physical exercise undertaken by men and women across the lifespan. Not surprisingly it mirrors the weight graph closely.

Sun cancers and melanoma are at epidemic levels for the white races, and these too take off at 40.

While patients may go to get their blood pressure, glucose and cholesterol checked, it is more usually acute illnesses that drive us to the doctor.

Section 2:

The Lists

Prioritized Lists
of
Prematurely Fatal Illnesses
or
Cause Premature Disabilities

Official Statistics

These lists are from Official Statistics for the USA, UK and Australia. It can be seen that there is a great concordance rate making them *applicable throughout the Western World.* Minor differences occur do due mainly to different national laws such as gun control.

These lists provide a valuable <u>guide</u> e.g. as can be seen in the USA Bureau of Statistics Survey of Disabilities, at age 18 to 24 years only 2.9% of the population had difficulty walking three city blocks, yet 11.3% of those between 45 and 64 years old had trouble rising to 31.7% for those over 65 years. These figures are not set in cement and vary from generation to generation, nation to nation and so on. But as a guide they reveal what we are likely to be "in for" and how we can take avoiding action. Walking speed has been shown to be directly linked to longevity. Resistance exercises are also good for us but in the same survey while only 2.3 % had trouble lifting 10 pound weights aged 18 to 44 21.8% had trouble when older than 65 years. The lessons to be taken from these surveys is to be conscious of walking quickly doing resistance training and attending to these other, mostly avoidable, disabilities of aging.

Disabilities may be approached in two different ways

1) **The actual disability e.g. Unable to turn on a tap**
2) **The causative condition e.g. arthritis**

Defined Age Groups per Country

For some reason, known only to statisticians, they all use different age groupings. While the USA groups below are the most widely used by their most reputable Authorities another (the US Census Bureau) uses the Australian age groups.

USA: 15-24, 26-34, 35-44, 45-54, 55-64, 55-74, 75+

UK: 20-34, 35-49, 50-64, 65-79, 80+

Australia: 15-24, 25-44, 45-64, 65-84, 84-94, 95+

Abbreviations: Some use "Statistician Speak" such as "Transport Accidents (land)" which I lump as Road Traffic Accidents (RTA) and "Unintentional Injuries" which I have listed as "Accidents". Elsewhere the standard medical abbreviations apply viz: Cardiovascular Disease = CVD, Metastatc Neoplasms = Cancer

Three Lists

There are three main Lists, but only two, which are relevant:
Each country has different systems of age-groups and not just simple decade by decade.

How To Use These Lists

For your age and sex, you can look up those potentially fatal and debilitating illnesses and take measures to avoid or prevent them. These are "The Missing Keys".

1. **Causes of Death by age and sex**

   We should all live to be over 80 years of age. If this is not achieved there are some illnesses or accidents that cause this premature demise. If then, these age specific illnesses are identified, avoidance or preventive measures can be instituted for each age group below 80 years.
   Males accounted for 62% of premature deaths.
   1 in 2 premature deaths were considered potentially avoidable.

2. **Causes of Disabilities by age and sex.**

   There are many illnesses that while they do not kill us effectively turn us into invalids e.g. a stroke may not be fatal but leave us paralysed down one side and unable to talk. Obviously preventing such disabilities is of prime focus and this again can best be achieved by consulting these Disability Lists.

   Due to improving medical care people are being saved from death and so disability survivors are increasing.

3. **Causes of Overall Deaths** - all ages - male and female.

   While they are of interest and listed below they are not of much help.

Age-Specific Analysis

Introduction

What illnesses affect you, for your age and sex as an individual, living in a First World country, are tabled herewith. If you study these age-group-specific tables you will identify those illnesses that you are most likely to encounter and which you should now take steps to avoid or minimize. How to do so is then documented.

Age-Specific Analysis

By examining these age-specific tables allows us to perform the most useful relevant tests. A cholesterol test may be done once in our 20s just to rule out any abnormality and, if normal, need not be repeated for some time. However, once we reach 40 it is a good idea to repeat it every 5 years or so even if it was originally normal.

Most serious illnesses seem to "take off" at age 40. Like the results of smoking (lung cancer and heart attacks) and the sun (skin wrinkles and cancer) this is not a sudden development but rather a process of long, chronic abuse. If we also abuse our arteries by overloading them with fats and high blood pressure, we don't have a "sudden" heart attack but one due to eating the wrong foods and not looking after ourselves. These Age-Specific Analyses then serve as harbingers, which, if we learn from them, can redirect our efforts away from the dangers.

These graphs and tables represent the illnesses, in order, which are most likely to disable us at our present age. Being disabled is usually the result of a serious condition that may have killed us but didn't, thus causing a permanent disability.

While most countries identify the Causes of Death for each age groups (which differ from country to country), few identify the illnesses or conditions that disable us, The best identification came from Australia in the 1990s when they even combined mortality and disablement in the same graphs in the same bar line:

The most helpful graphs combined Causes of Disabilities with Causes of Deaths for each age group and sex. This showed the relationship between the two as in the example graph below. Here it can be seen how malignant neoplasms (cancer) causes more premature deaths than Disabilities when compared to Cardiovascular Disease which at the age this graph represents, causes more overall Premature health problems. Whereas Musculoskeletal diseases cause far more Disabilities than Deaths (so this graph must be for a relatively younger person).

Unfortunately these graphs are not done anymore but are included as they still provide the best visual comparisons and information.

Don't be put off with the statistician-speak of YLD, YLL and DALYS. All we need to know is that:

Light bar = Disability

Dark bar = Premature death by the same illness

Explanation of Combination Graph

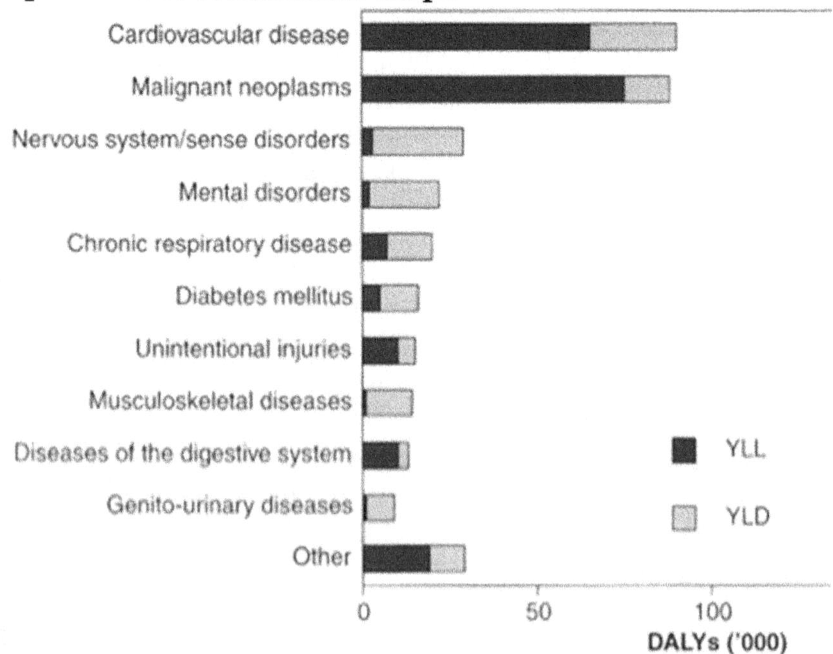

Years lost to disabilities are always more than from premature deaths.

The DALY is the combination of both = total years of healthy life lost.

How to Use These Graphs and Lists

Unfortunately, as noted, these combined graphs of mortality and disabilities are no longer provided. Most graphs are now only for mortality but, nevertheless, provide great information because as can be seen from these combined graphs Premature Deaths and Disabilities often shadow each other.

The combined graphs are provided at the end of each age group.

Male and Female are in separated sections. Identify which section you want. The Male section is first.

Find the Table/Graph for your age and sex and see what illnesses are most likely to disable (and kill) you, then take diagnostic and preventive action.

After each age group for each sex there is an analysis as to what to do to prevent these illnesses.

Many of the illnesses and conditions (like blood pressure, high cholesterol and early cancers) have no symptoms. Prioritizing them allows for specific focus, with the appropriate investigations and preventive measures, rather than the previous generalized, one-size-fits-all recommendations. By identifying your age and sex you will know exactly what to focus upon.

The statistics and data are relevant for all First World countries based on US, UK and Australian data.

Hence if you are a 45- to 54-year-old female, you are most likely to die from breast cancer in the United States and United Kingdom, but from Coronary Artery Disease (CAD) if Australian.

Then run down the list and see what others, in order, are most likely to kill you.

Also look ahead at the next decade.

These two decades, your present and next decades, give you the conditions you must now seek to avoid immediately, and alert you to take preventive measures for the future. An American 45–54-year-old female is most likely to die from breast cancer, then from coronary artery disease, lung cancer and poisoning. This then alerts a woman in this age bracket to get screened for breast cancer, heart disease, lung cancer; while poisoning may mean a risk of depression/suicide. Just for these four risks, the following measures would then seem mandatory and preventive: a breast examination and a mammogram, a cardiovascular check including serum lipids (LDL) and ECG/EKG, blood pressure check, chest x-ray, and ceasing smoking, plus seeking help if depressed. After all, blood pressure and lipids can be treated by better nutrition and exercise or medications; breast cancer if diagnosed early is usually curable; and lung cancer is overwhelmingly caused by smoking—so stop now! Depression also responds to treatment. But all these require you to be aware of what illnesses you are most likely to encounter, and to actively seek screening/diagnosis, and to then take immediate and long-term preventive action or get treatment. This systematic and logical plan of attack is applicable to all of us, for each decade and each sex.

The overall data (for all ages combined) is included for interest only; it highlights that heart or cardiovascular disease is the overall number-one killer for essentially all First World nations.

Conclusions

These tables provide the essential statistical evidence prioritizing the most serious illnesses. Later how to avoid or diagnose and cure them is addressed. Fourteen or more of these “Top 21” causes of death or disabilities are arguably preventable or able to be diagnosed early enough to effect a cure.

Heart disease is our overall number-one killer and cause of us being disabled. Combined with the other main circulatory problems of cerebrovascular disease (strokes) and other heart disorders, they are massively, by far and away, worse than the next health problem.

It is therefore obvious we should make cardiovascular disease our main prevention priority.

NOTE: Alzheimer's is not an actual "cause of death." The most common cause of death in individuals with advanced Alzheimer's disease is an intercurrent infection, mostly pneumonia—as Sir William Osler noted, "Pneumonia may well be called the friend of the aged." An intercurrent infection is the almost inevitable consequence of advanced dementia because of impairment of immune function and aspiration, inability to ambulate, and incontinence.

Emergency Signs and Prevention

These lists alert us to the most likely illnesses that occur for our age. This book also provides the best evidenced advice on how to avoid them. However, the other essential is recognizing any acute and potentially serious symptoms and signs if and when they occur. Early medical attention results in the best outcomes. When I ran the Coronary Care Unit the greatest delay in patients being admitted occurred because they "didn't want to bother anyone." The average delay, from memory, was some four to six hours before they called the ambulance, and in those days the ambulance response time was slower. Today, however, while people may still "not want to bother anyone," most are either in denial or don't recognize their symptoms as being potentially serious.

The following are Emergency Signs.

If you experience any of these, get checked out *immediately:*

1. Chest pain like indigestion that wont go away. This is a heart attack until proven otherwise.
2. FAST: Face – drooping; Arms – weakness; Speech – slurred, difficult; Time – urgent.
3. Momentary loss of vision. This may be a Transient Ischaemic Attack warning of a Stroke.
4. Chronic cough especially in smokers.
5. Change in bowel habit.
6. Unexplained loss of weight or tiredness.
7. Nocturia (having to get up to void at night).
8. Intermenstrual bleeding.

13. Causes of Premature Death by Age and Sex (USA, UK, Australia)

UPDATE APRIL 2017: OBESITY THE BIGGEST CAUSE OF PREMATURE DEATH

Obesity is the top cause of a shortened life span ahead of diabetes, tobacco use, high blood pressure and high cholesterol, according to the Cleveland Clinic and New York University School of Medicine.

Obesity resulted in as much as 47% more life-years lost than tobacco, and tobacco was as life-shortening as high blood pressure.

These preliminary results continue to highlight the importance of weight loss, diabetes management and healthy eating with diabetes, high blood pressure and high cholesterol all able to be treated.

TOP 10 CAUSES OF DEATH

	USA 2014	UK 2013	Australia 2015
1	Heart disease	Heart disease	Heart disease
2	Cancer	Lung cancer	DementiaAlzheim.
3	Ch low respiratory diseases	Dementia Alzheimer's	Cerebrovascular disease
4	Unintentional injuries	Emphysema/bronchitis	Trachea, bronchus lung cancer
5	Cerebrovascular diseases	Cerebrovascular diseases	Chronic lower respiratory diseases
6	Alzheimer's D.	Flu/pneumonia	Diabetes
7	Diabetes mellitus	Prostate cancer	Colon cancer
8	Influenza and pneumonia	Bowel cancer	Blood, lymph cancer (leukaemia)
9	Kidney disease	Lymphoid cancer	Heart failure
0	Suicide	Liver disease	Diseases of the urinary system

These lists should be used as an overall - not age specific - guide.

It can be seen these and all first world countries share the same Top 10.

Death after the age of 80 years is the ambition and is not "Premature".

USA Overall Causes Of Death

Latest Figures[55]

The age-adjusted death rate in the United States hit an all-time low in 2014, at 724.6 deaths per 100,000, down 1% from 2013. Heart disease and cancer were still the top two causes of death in the United States in 2014, according to new data from the National Center for Health Statistics published June 30 in *National Vital Statistics Reports*.

The top 10 causes of death in 2014 were as follows:

1. Heart disease (23.4% of all deaths)
2. Cancer (22.5%)
3. Chronic lower respiratory diseases (5.6%)
4. Accidents (unintentional injuries; 5.2%)
5. Cerebrovascular diseases (5.1%)
6. Alzheimer's disease (3.6%)
7. Diabetes mellitus (2.9%)
8. Influenza and pneumonia (2.1%)
9. Nephritis, nephrotic syndrome, and nephrosis (1.8%)
10. Intentional self-harm (suicide; 1.6%).

Together these 10 causes of death accounted for 74% of all deaths in the United States. They are unchanged from the top 10 causes of death in 2013.

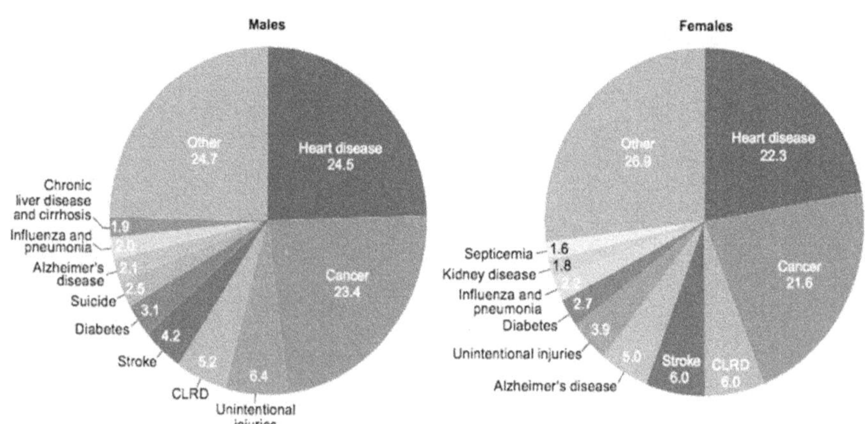

NOTES: CLRD is Chronic lower respiratory diseases. Values show percentage of total deaths.
SOURCE: NCHS, National Vital Statistics System, Mortality.

Distribution % the 10 leading causes of death, by age USA 2014

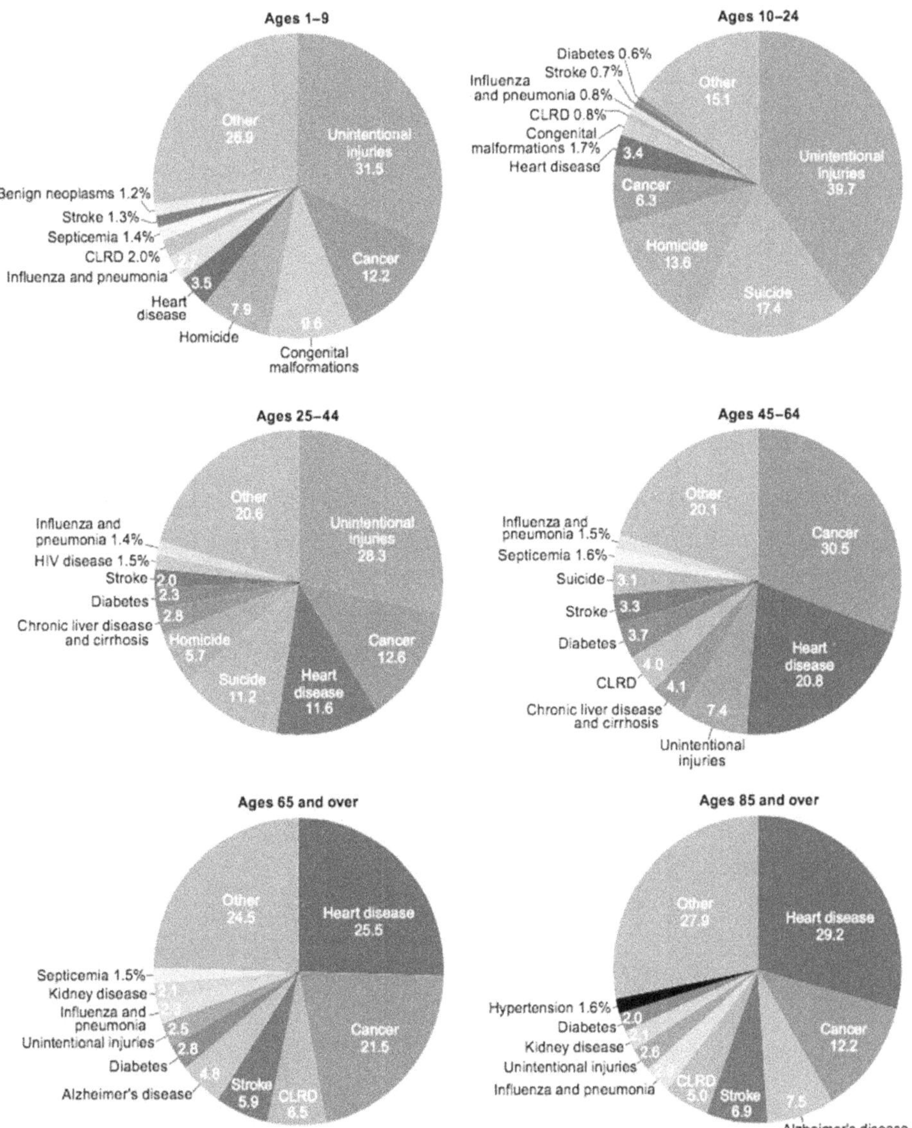

NOTES: CLRD is Chronic lower respiratory diseases; HIV is Human immunodeficiency virus. Values show percentage of total deaths. SOURCE: NCHS, National Vital Statistics System, Mortality.

U.K.
Leading causes of deaths registered in England and Wales, 2013

1. Heart disease
2. Lung cancer
3. Dementia andAlzheimer's
4. Emphysema/bronchitis
5. Cerebrovasculardiseases
6. Flu/pneumonia
7. Prostate cancer
8. Bowel cancer
9. Lymphoidcancer
10. Liver disease
11. Throatcancer
12. Suicide
13. Urinarydisease
14. Pancreaticcancer
15. Heart failure

The following figures and graphs are from the UK Office for National Statistics as %. They are, like those for the USA above, here not only for interest but to see the evolution and changes as to what illnesses we encounter as we grow older.

Top 5 leading causes of death 2015 England and Wales
5-19 years

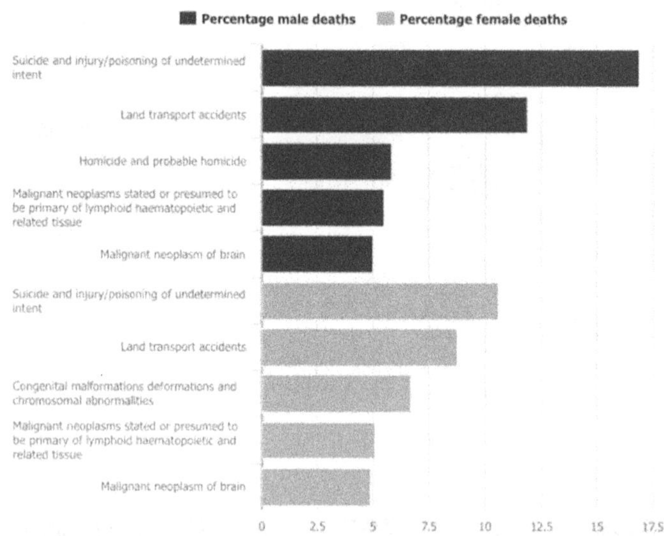

20-34 years

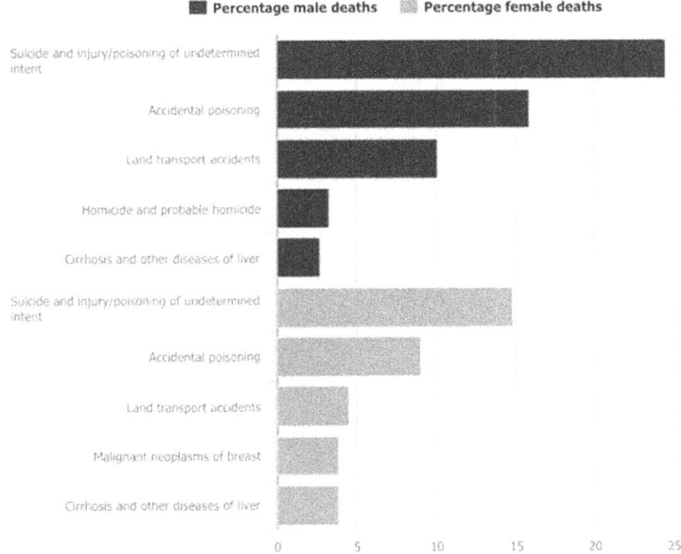

35 49 Years

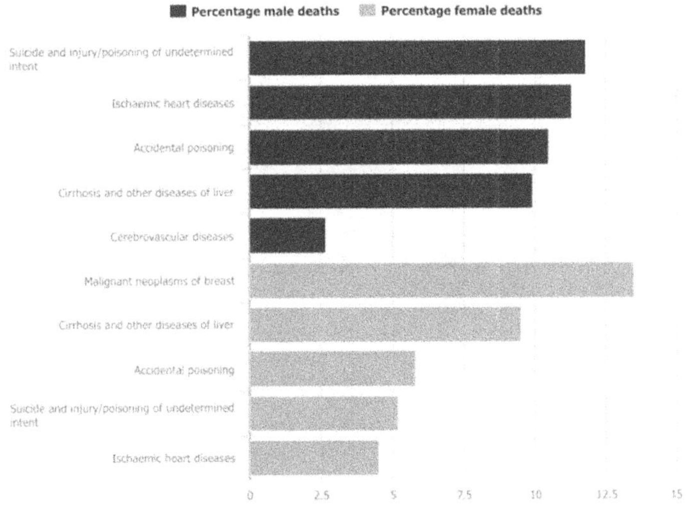

55-64 years

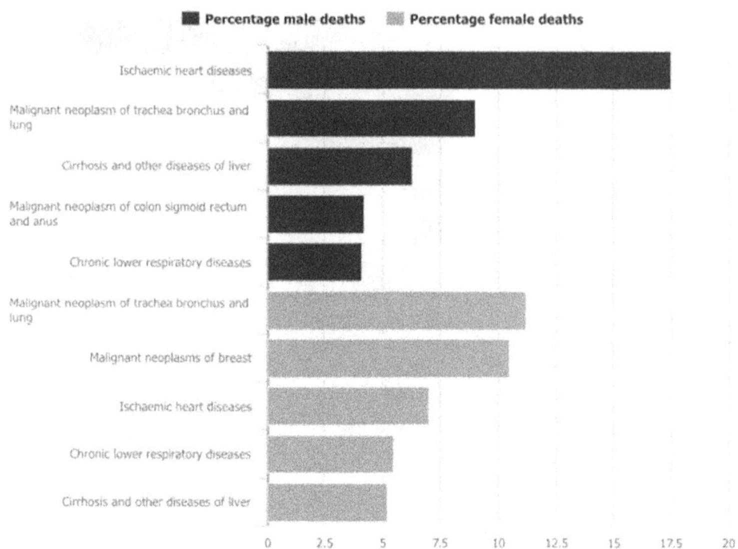

65-79 years

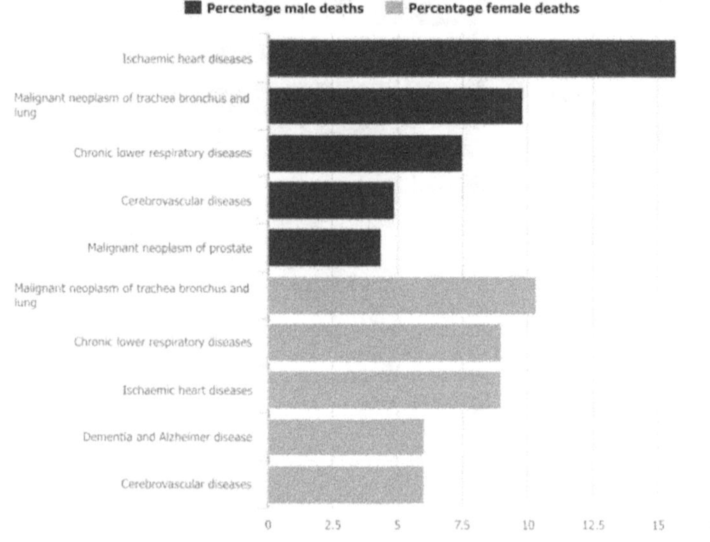

14. Causes of Premature Disabilities by Age and Sex (USA, UK, Australia)

Disabilities

Obviously, this category is broad and constantly shifting, so exact statistics are hard to come by, but the data from our most reliable sources is surprising. The Centers for Disease Control and Prevention estimates that one in five adults in the United States is living with a disability. The National Organization on Disability says there are 56 million disabled people. Indeed, people with disabilities are the largest minority group in the United States, and as new disability categories such as neurodiversity, psychiatric disabilities, disabilities of aging and learning disabilities emerge and grow, so does that percentage. These statistics are applicable to all first world countries and average 20% (one in five) of the population, increasing with age.

The three most common causes of disability in the USA continued to be arthritis or rheumatism, back or spine problems and heart trouble. Women (24.4%) had a significantly higher prevalence of disability compared with men (19.1%) at all ages. For both sexes, the prevalence of disability doubled in successive age groups (18--44 years, 11.0%; 45--64 years, 23.9%; and ≥65 years, 51.8%)

What Are Disabilities

Two aspects

1. **Actual Practical Impediment**
2. **Actual Medical Causative Conditions**

The following lists not only show the progression of various Disabilities with age but those we are likely to encounter. Many of these are unvoiced: People are not likely to talk as to how they now find difficulty bathing but from age 18 years to 65 years it has become x 13 times more difficult! This was brought home to me when a 75 year old patient complained how he "could no longer wipe his bottom" - hardly something he is going to tell his friends but, more's the point, something he could have avoided had he known, as you can now, what Disabilities we are in for.

Look at the 18 year old columns and then the 65 years old column and see what Disabilities show the greatest increases: Hearing, Walking three city Blocks, Lifting 10 pounds, Getting out of a chair, Bathing, Taking care of money, Preparing meals or Light housework.

Most, if not all of these can be avoided or considerably minimized. Each should now be addressed to assess your future potential predicaments and prevention or minimization tactics now started.

As examples, I had a great friend who was twice the British Actor of the Year and a ferocious tennis competitor even though he was 15 years my senior. We would play five sets of tennis (and not "tip and giggle" but flat strap). One year he showed me how he was now doing yoga and could grab both hands behind his back with one over his shoulder and the other behind his waist. I am sure he had no trouble wiping his bottom and lived working to 89 years of age.

My neighbor uses noisy mowers and brush-cutters but doesn't wear ear-muffs. Elsewhere I noted my Rock Drummer friend and the hoons at the traffic lights with their 12 surround speakers lifting their car into the ear with each beat...all destined for hearing losses but all preventable.

I am surprised at the fall off in exercise capacity which I can only think is due to not exercising except, if we look at the next table as to the Actual Medical Causes it can be seen that Arthritis, Spine and heart troubles are the big three which may restrict some, but not all, such exercises.

It is all in the next two tables for you to ponder your future...and take avoiding or preventive action.

If you know what you are likely to encounter you can avoid, prevent or minimize them.

1. Actual Practical Impediment

Most of us may be unaware of just what Disabilities are or how they impact on lives as the following reveal:

Estimated number* and percentage of civilian noninstitutionalized adults aged ≥18 years with self-reported disabilities, by age group --- United States, 2005

	% 18 - 44 yrs	**% 45 - 64 yrs**	**→% 65 (+) yrs**
Difficulty with specified functional activities	6.3	19.4	47.5
Seeing words/letters in newsprint	1.3	3.8	
Hearing normal conversation	1.1	3.6	11.2
Having speech understood	0.8	1.1	2.1
Walking three city blocks	2.9	11.3	31.7
Climbing a flight of stairs	2.8	11.4	30.2
Grasping objects	1.0	4.2	8.2
Lifting/Carrying 10 lbs	2.3	7.8	21.8
Difficulty with activities of daily living	1.0	4.1	12.5
Getting around inside home	0.4	1.8	6.4
Getting in/out of bed/chair	0.6	2.7	7.5
Bathing	0.6	2.2	7.9
Dressing	0.5	1.7	5.3
Eating	0.2	0.6	2.1
Toileting	0.3	1.0	3.6
Difficulty with instrumental activities of daily living	2.2	6.0	19.1
Getting around outside of home	1.1	3.8	
Taking care of money and bills	1.1	1.7	7.4
Preparing meals	0.8	1.8	8.0
Doing light housework	0.9	3.2	9.9
Managing prescriptions	0.7	1.6	6.2
Using the telephone	0.4	0.8	4.6

Reporting of selected impairments	5.6	6.9	8.1
A learning disability	2.2	1.3	0.6
Mental retardation	0.7	0.4	0.3
Other developmental disability	0.4	0.2	0.1
Alzheimer's disease/senility/dementia	0.3	0.6	3.8
Other mental/emotional disability	3.5	5.6	5.6
Use of assistive aid	1.0	4.6	19.2
Wheelchair	0.4	1.3	5.2
Cane, crutches, or walker	0.8	4.2	17.9
Limitation in ability to work around the house	3.5	10.7	20.3
Limitation in ability to work at a job or business**	4.5	11.3	

2. Actual Medical Causative Conditions

Main cause of disability among civilian non-institutionalized U.S.adults aged ≥18 years with self-reported disabilities

	Total	**Men**	**Women**
Conditions	**%**	**%**	**%**
Arthritis or rheumatism	19.0	11.5	24.3
Back or spine problems	16.8	16.9	16.8
Heart trouble	6.6	8.4	5.4
Lung or respiratory problem	4.9	4.9	4.9
Mental or emotional problem	4.9	5.2	4.6
Diabetes	4.5	4.8	4.2
Deafness or hearing problem	4.2	6.8	2.4
Stiffness or deformity of limbs/ extremities	3.6	3.6	3.7

Blindness or vision problem	3.2	3.9	2.8
Stroke	2.4	3.1	1.9
Cancer	2.2	2.4	2.1
Broken bone/fracture	2.1	1.9	2.3
High blood pressure	1.9	1.6	2.1
Mental retardation	1.5	1.7	1.3
Senility/Dementia/Alzheimer's	1.2	1.0	1.3
Head or spinal cord injury	1.1	1.5	0.9
Learning disability	1.1	1.6	0.7
Kidney problems	0.9	1.2	0.7
Stomach/Digestive problems	0.8	0.7	0.8
Paralysis of any kind	0.6	0.7	0.5
Epilepsy	0.6	0.6	0.6
Hernia or rupture	0.5	0.6	0.5
Cerebral palsy	0.5	0.8	0.3
Missing limbs/extremities	0.5	0.8	0.2
Alcohol or drug problem	0.4	0.8	0.2
Tumor/Cyst/Growth	0.3	0.2	0.3
Thyroid problems	0.2	0.1	0.3
AIDS or AIDS-related	0.2	0.2	0.2
Speech disorder	0.2	0.1	0.2
Other	12.9	12.1	13.5
Total*	**100.0**	**100.0**	**100.0**

SOURCE: U.S. Census Bureau, 2004 Survey of Income and Program Participation, 2005.

Over 1 in 4 of today's 20 year-olds will become disabled before they retire.

Over 37 million Americans are classified as disabled; about 12% of the total population. More than 50% of those disabled Americans are in their working years, from 18-64..

USA Overall Causes Of Disability in Men[72]

Disability	% Affected
Back or spinal problems	16.9
Arthritis or Rheumatism	11.5
Heart trouble	8.4
Deafness or impeded hearing	6.6
Mental or emotional problems	5.2
Lung or respiratory problems	4.9
Diabetes	4.8
Vision problems or blindness	3.9
Stiffness or deformity of limbs	3.6
Stroke	3.1
Cancer	2.4
Fractures – broken bones	1.9

By 2030, and that's closer than we think, the number of U.S. adults aged ≥65 years will approximately double from current numbers to about 71 million. The implications of this growing number of older adults include unprecedented demands on public health and senior services and the nation's health-care system. For example, greater numbers of trained professionals will be needed to expand the reach of effective community-based programs to mitigate the effects of disability. Modifiable lifestyle characteristics (e.g., physical inactivity, obesity, and tobacco use) are major contributors to the most common causes of disability, and sometimes stem from a primary disabling condition. Widespread use of effective, population-based approaches to increase physical activity, reduce obesity and tobacco use, and provide health promotion education programs for persons with an existing disability can reduce the incidence of various associated chronic conditions, prevent some disabilities, and reduce the severity of others. Regular physical activity is effective in reducing morbidity resulting from heart disease and reducing or eliminating multiple associated risk factors. Physical activity also has been shown to prevent episodes of back problems, reduce pain, improve physical function, and delay disability among adults with arthritis. Health-care providers should consider early referral to interventions that can prevent or reduce severity of disability for patients at high risk for disability (e.g., women and persons with chronic musculoskeletal conditions).[6]

People across the world are living longer but often spending more time in ill health, as rates of non-fatal diseases and injuries decline more slowly than death rates, according to a new analysis of 301 diseases and injuries in 188 countries, many in the Third World with malaria, poor hygiene, infected water and so on.[65] Rates of disability are declining much more slowly than death rates; for example, while increases in rates of diabetes have been substantial, rising by around 43% over the past 23 years, death rates from diabetes increased by only 9%.[66]

Just one in 20 people worldwide (4.3%) had no health problems in 2013, with a third of the world's population (2.3 billion individuals) experiencing more than five ailments. In the past 23 years, the leading causes of health loss have hardly changed. Low back pain, depression, iron-deficiency anemia, neck pain, and age-related hearing loss resulted in the largest overall health loss worldwide. In 2013, musculoskeletal disorders (i.e., mainly low back pain, neck pain, and arthritis) and mental and substance abuse disorders (predominantly depression, anxiety, and drug and alcohol use disorders) accounted for almost half of all health loss worldwide.

The recent improvement in statistics helps identify what are cumbersomely labeled "Non-Fatal Burdens of Disease" (NFBD). I think we can just call them "Burdens" as it's hard to conceive a burden if we are dead.

It would seem all of us are destined to be burdened in some way in our final years. These new statistics allow construction of a logical, systematic and focused preventive or minimization plan.

What disables or kills us at 25 is different from when we are 60. These disabling illnesses are also often different for men and women. Alcohol and cars figure prominently in the tables for young men, but not

---

[6] Prevalence and Most Common Causes of Disability Among Adults --- United States, 2005. CDC Bureau of Satistics MMWR Report May 1 2009/58(16);421-426

for women; and obviously men hardly get any breast cancer. As will be seen, the disability invariably contributes to the person's death, but not always.

The whole thrust of this **Missing Keys** is to identify, avoid or minimize these disabilities both in severity and duration, in combination with Successful Aging, Nutrition, Exercise and Weight Plans so as to Live Longest.

One recent study reported that Americans are living longer but in poorer health. (This is contradicted below). The analysis of US vital statistics of life expectancy trends and disability rates in a 40-year period, from 1970 to 2010, found that the average total lifespan increased for men and women in those 40 years, but so did the proportion of time spent living with a disability.

In the United States increasing longevity is not necessarily indicative of good health; most age groups are now living longer, but with a disability or other health problem increasing the length of a poor-quality life more than a good-quality life.

The Baby Boomer generation, which is now reaching old age, is not seeing improvements in health similar to the older groups that went before them. Only for people aged 65 and older was there a "compression of morbidity"—a reduction in the proportion of years spent with disability or ill health.

Clearly, there is a need to maintain health and reduce disability at younger ages to have meaningful compression of morbidity across the age ranges.

The average lifespan for men increased by 9.2 years to 76.2 years. The number of years they live with a disability increased by 4.7 years, while the number of years spent disability-free increased by 4.5 years.

American women have not done as well as American men in terms of improving health in recent decades. Their average lifespan increased by 6.4 years to 81 years. The number of years that women spend with a disability increased by 3.6 years, exceeding the increase in women's disability-free life (2.7 years).

Different factors may affect disability at different ages. For instance, younger populations may have had an increase in disability because of a greater emphasis on mental health, increased diagnoses of autism spectrum and attention deficit hyperactivity disorders, and changes in drug use.[67]

However, in contrast to the above, the latest study shows that the increase in life expectancy in the past two decades has been accompanied by an even greater increase in life years free of disability, which, as you will see, is the main aim of this game - Compression of Morbidity (Sicker shorter, healthier longer).

The study found that in 1992, the life expectancy of the average 65-year-old was 17.5 years, 8.9 of which were free from disability. By 2008, total life expectancy had risen to 18.8 years. In addition to the overall increase, the number of disability-free years increased, from 8.9 to 10.7, while the number of disabled years fell, from 8.6 to 8.1in contrast to the above. Driving those changes were cardiovascular health and vision treatment, with an incredibly dramatic decline in deaths and disabilities from heart disease and heart failure as the result of people smoking less and better diet. But it was estimated that as much as half of the improvement is because of medical care, especially statin drug treatment, which is both preventing heart attacks and improving people's recovery. Much of the improvement in vision health is due to improved quicker and cheaper treatment of cataracts.[68]

The above examples show what can be done, but the improvement can still be much better, and arguably with much fewer medications, by following the ***Live Longest*** advice.

Multiple Chronic Conditions – Disabilities
Approximately 25% of U.S. adults have diagnoses of MCC. Data from the 2014 National Health Interview Survey (NHIS) were used to estimate prevalence of MCC (defined as two or more of 10 diagnosed chronic conditions) for each U.S. state and region by age and sex. Adults who reported a diagnosis of two or more of the following selected conditions were categorized as having MCC: arthritis, asthma, cancer, chronic obstructive pulmonary disease (COPD), coronary heart disease, diabetes, hepatitis, hypertension, stroke, or weak or failing kidneys. Significant state and regional variation in MCC prevalence was found, with state-level estimates ranging from 19.0% in Colorado to 38.2% in Kentucky. MCC prevalence also varied by region.[70]

Chances of becoming disabled: >40% if overweight and smoking
A typical female, age 35, 5'4", 125 pounds, non-smoker, who works mostly an office job, with some outdoor physical responsibilities, and who leads a healthy lifestyle has the following risks:

A 24% chance of becoming disabled for 3 months or longer during her working career, with a 38% chance that the disability would last 5 years or longer and with the average disability for someone like her lasting 82 months.

If this same person used tobacco and weighed 160 pounds, the risk would increase to a 41% chance of becoming disabled for 3 months or longer.

A typical male, age 35, 5'10", 170 pounds, non-smoker, who works an office job, with some outdoor physical responsibilities, and who leads a healthy lifestyle has the following risks:

A 21% chance of becoming disabled for 3 months or longer during his working career, with a 38% chance that the disability would last 5 years or longer and with the average disability for someone like him lasting 82 months.

If this same person used tobacco and weighed 210 pounds, the risk would increase to a 45% chance of becoming disabled for 3 months or longer.

CDA's PDQ disability risk calculator

UK

There are 12.9 million disabled people in the UK.

- 7 per cent of children are disabled
- 17 per cent of working age adults are disabled
- 45 per cent of pension age adults are disabled

The most commonly reported impairments by disabled people are:

- Mobility (53%)
- Stamina, breathing, fatigue (39%)
- Dexterity (29%).

Land transport accidents leading cause of death for 5-19 year olds

The leading cause of death for both males and females aged 5-19 was land transport accidents, accounting for 13% of deaths at this age group. This was more common among males than females. Worldwide, males under the age of 25 are almost three times more likely to be killed in a car crash than females of the same age. Suicide is also one of the leading causes of death among this age group; the 2nd leading cause of death of males (112 deaths) and 6th for females (23 deaths).

Suicide and accidental poisoning leading cause of death for 20-34 year olds

Suicide (including injury/poisoning of undetermined intent) was the leading cause of death for 20-34 year olds (24% of men and 12% of women). Factors that could lead to these deaths include: traumatic experiences, lifestyle choices such as drug or alcohol misuse, job insecurity and relationship problems. For both sexes, accidental poisoning is also a highly common cause of death, followed by land transport accidents.

Breast cancer leading cause of death for 35-49 year old women

Suicide remains the leading cause of death for men aged 35-49, accounting for 13% of deaths. Breast cancer is the leading cause of death among women in this age group, accounting for 14% of deaths. However, it is the leading cause because women in this age group are relatively healthy and are therefore less likely to die of other causes. Breast cancer deaths in women aged 15-49 years only account for around 10% of all female breast cancer deaths.

Heart disease leading cause of death for men aged 50 and over

For those aged 50 and over, the leading causes of death for both men and women were long-term diseases and conditions. Cancer of the trachea, bronchus and lung is the number one cause for women aged 50-64, accounting for 11% of deaths in this group. Breast cancer is the 2nd leading cause of death for 50-64 year old women, accounting for 11% of deaths in this age group. Heart diseases are the leading cause of death for men aged 50 and over. Lifestyle choices and other conditions can lead to heart disease such as: smoking, high cholesterol, high blood pressure and diabetes.

Dementia and Alzheimer's leading cause of death for women over 80

Dementia and Alzheimer's disease was the leading cause of death for women over 80 accounting for 17% of deaths and was the second leading cause for men causing 11% of deaths in this age group. Deaths from dementia and Alzheimer's disease are increasing as people live longer, and are more common in women as women live longer than men. The leading cause of death for men in this age group was ischaemic heart disease accounting for 15% of deaths, this was the second leading cause for women causing 11% of deaths In the UK around 6% of children are disabled, compared to 16% of working age adults and 45% of adults over State Pension age.

AUSTRALIA

In Australia 18.5% reported having a disability in 2009, according to the results of the Survey of Disability, Ageing and Carers (SDAC). For the purposes of SDAC, disability is defined as any limitation, restriction or impairment which restricts everyday activities and has lasted or is likely to last for at least six months. Examples range from loss of sight that is not corrected by glasses, to arthritis which causes difficulty dressing, to advanced dementia that requires constant help and supervision. Males and females were similarly affected by disability (18% and 19% respectively)

Leading single causes of burden of disease and injury in men by age

Condition	DALYs	Per cent of total
25–44 years		
Suicide and self-inflicted injuries	23,296	10.3
Depression	16,827	7.4
Road traffic accidents	14,929	6.6
Alcohol dependence and harmful use	13,026	5.8
HIV/AIDS	10,250	4.5
All causes total	**225,873**	
45–64 years		
Ischaemic heart disease	57,521	16.7
Lung cancer	22,509	6.5
Chronic obstructive pulmonary disease	16,999	4.9
Hearing loss	15,861	4.6
Diabetes mellitus	15,711	4.6
All causes total	**345,095**	
65 years and over		
Ischaemic heart disease	113,681	21.7
Stroke	45,111	8.6
Lung cancer	36,206	6.9
Chronic obstructive pulmonary disease	30,348	5.8
Alzheimer's disease and other dementias	27,804	5.3
All causes total	**523,774**	

Note: These are the order of conditions which make someone an disabled but not that for premature deaths. However they are often the same.

Two Decade Analysis Reveals Risk Factors Are on the Rise Despite Greater Awareness

Despite increased understanding of heart disease risk factors and the need for preventive lifestyle changes, patients suffering the most severe type of heart attack (ST-elevation myocardial infarction, or STEMI) have become younger, more obese and more likely to have preventable risk factors such as smoking, high blood pressure, diabetes and chronic obstructive pulmonary disease.[73]

Whereas in 1999, cardiovascular disease (CVD) excluding stroke was the main cause of death in all US states except Alaska, 14 years later, deaths from cancer surpassed those from CVD in almost half of the states, a new study reports.[74]

About half of the dramatic reduction in heart-disease mortality can be attributed to better treatments such as revascularization, and about half to reductions in risk factors such as smoking, cholesterol, and blood pressure, but not BMI or diabetes.[75]

Conditions Patients Believe to be Worse Than Death

While death may be considered the ultimate "adverse outcome" by doctors, many patients with serious illness consider some debilitating conditions to be even worse than death (University of Pennsylvania).

The responses showed that six conditions were rated as bad or worse than death by a significant proportion of patients:

1. Bowel and bladder incontinence
2. Relying on a breathing machine to live
3. Being unable to get out of bed
4. Being confused all the time
5. Having to rely on a feeding tube to live
6. Needing care all the time

Four more conditions that were rated as somewhat better than death were: 7. living in a nursing home, 8. being at home all day, 9. being in moderate pain all the time, and 10.being in a wheelchair.[69]

15. Men Under 24 years

USA Males 20-24	UK Males 5 - 19 yrs	Australia 15-24
Unintentional injuries 42.7%	Transport Accidents (Land)	Suicide
Suicide 18.8%	Suicide	Land Transport Accidents
Homicide 16.8%	Homicide	Accidental Poisoning
Cancer 4.2%	Lymphoid Cancer	Assault
Heart Disease 3.0%	Congenital Defects	Event of undetermined intent
Birth Defects 0.8%	Cerebral Palsy / Paralytic Syndromes	
Diabetes 0.6%	Brain Cancer	
Flu & Pneumonia 0.5%	Accidental Poisoning	
Ch Lower Respiratory D	Accidental threats to breathing	
Stroke 0.5%	Emphysema / Bronchitis	

Although we know that high-risk behavior is common in young men and leads to injuries and deaths, the data on “fun activities” is not well known.

A study of youth and adolescents 5–19 years of age who were treated in US emergency departments (EDs) found that over a 19-year period, there were an average of 176 a day for skateboarding-related injuries.[71]

Quad bikes are the greatest cause of injury and deaths on farms.

Diving into shallow water, drugs, alcohol and driving too fast are perhaps better known.

Many of these are a matter of “boys being boys,” but the risks are underestimated and dangerous.

What To Do

As can be seen in the next age group "Drugs, Booze and Testosterone" are also manifesting here in this age group. It is a too-often deadly combination as youth experiments and pushes the boundaries.

Parental control can give way to guidance and advice but this age group consider themselves "bullet proof" and only the death of a close friend may alert them to modify their high-risk behaviors.

Sport has been a traditional outlet to attenuate the aggression that testosterone brings.

Suicide figures prominently and any signs of with-drawl, depression or "problems" must be acted on urgently.

Homicide would seem inexorably linked to liberal gun laws.

16. Men 25–34 (44) years

" Drugs, Booze and Testosterone"

Drugs, Booze and Testosterone

Drugs, booze and testosterone account for 70% of all deaths and disabilities in this age group, which is where to focus.

CAUSES OF DEATHS

	USA 25 -34 yrs	**UK 20 - 34 yrs**	**Australia 25 -44**
1	RTA	Suicide	Suicide
2	Homocide	Accidental Poisoning	Accidents
3	Suicide	RTA	Cancer
4	Poisoning	Homocide	Cardiovascular Disease
5	Other Injuries	Liver Disease	Infections / Parasitic Diseases
6	Drownings	Epilepsy	Mental Disorders
7	Endocrine Disorders	Heart Disease	Others
8	Congenital Abnormalities	Brain Cancer	Nervous System Disorders
9	Inflammatory / Heart	Lynphoid Cancer	Digestive System disorders
10	Leukemia	Cerebrovascular Disease	Ch Respiratory Disease

EVIDENCED PREVALENCE (in order)	**PREVENTIVE MEASURES**
1. Drugs & Booze – 38% Depression	Consider all males in this age group as substance abusers until proven otherwise. Warn and advise. Watch for depression—suicide.
2. Homicide (USA / UK)	Access to guns is the problem.
3. RTA / Accidents – 15%	Fast cars, testosterone and booze. Again, advice and counseling. Motor Bikes are very dangerous: 5% of vehicles but 25% of MVAs.
4. Suicide – 12%	Heightened awareness that this age group is at risk. Early diagnosis, support, advice +- antidepressants.
5. Cancer	Not as common as above but smoking and processed foods promote. Alert for change of bowel habit, change in behavior, smoker's cough.

EVIDENCED PREVALENCE (in order)	PREVENTIVE MEASURES
6. CVS	Shortness of breath on effort, chest pain. Screen. Better nutrition.
7. Infections	Cause. Overseas travel prophylaxis.
8. Chronic Respiratory Diseases	Asthma/emphysema. Cease smoking. Treat aggressively.
9. Musculoskeletal Diseases – Back Pain	Back pain starts at 20. Lifting advice. No strong-man show off. Bend knees.
10. Nervous Sys Multiple Sclerosis	No preventive measures as yet.
11. Digestive System	Heartburn: Lose weight, stop smoking, reduce booze, avoid PPIs. Investigate any others.

As a group the greatest cause of disabilities in this 25–44-year-old age group for men is **mental disorders,** which in turn are mainly due to **substance abuse—alcohol and illicit drugs—(38%)** and **depression (27%)** causing disability rather than premature deaths. In fact deaths in this first group have the lowest ratio to disabilities in the top six causes. Knowing that drugs, substance abuse and depression cause so many problems may facilitate an earlier diagnosis. Today it would seem naïve not to suspect substance abuse, which may also be a contributor to depression. Getting on the front foot and aggressively treating rather than suspecting depression is also arguably warranted.

Unintentional Injuries are second and *contribute more to death than disabilities* (as do the next five causes). They account for 15.5%, of which almost half are from road traffic accidents (RTA). This group represents the testosterone-fueled, high-risk behavior group—smoking, drinking, "never thinking of tomorrow," experimenting, showing off, driving too fast. The best prevention is to start early with advice, warnings, defensive driving courses and even a visit to the spinal injuries unit if the message isn't getting through. Dietary advice should have started as well. Motorbikes account for 5% of vehicles but 25% of accidents. Skate Boards and Mountain Biking take an increasing toll.

Intentional Injuries come third, making up some 12% of the total. Breaking down such injuries, 85% are due to suicide or self-inflicted injuries.

However, the largest *single* cause of disease and injury burden in this age group is suicide and self-inflicted injuries, at 10.3%; then depression (7.4%), road traffic accidents (6.6%), alcohol dependence/misuse (5.8%), HIV/AIDS (4.5%).

The message here is to get on the front foot and proactively assume depression and offer support, intervention and treatment to prevent suicide or attempted suicide. This, I feel, cannot be over-emphasized.

In the United States, due to their liberal gun laws, homicide is high on the list; but it is high also in the United Kingdom.

Cancer or malignant neoplasms are next, with brain cancers more common than most of us think; these are invariably fatal. Again, early diagnosis offers the best hope. Watch for any change of behavior. These changes may be subtle but should not be ignored. Headaches are not often a symptom but again should not be ignored; while paralysis or altered movement is an advanced sign. Cancer of the colon (CAC) is another we don't really associate with young men, but there are some famous young widows whose husbands died from CAC. Unexplained loss of weight, change of bowel habit, passing mucus, slime or blood, and undue fatigue are symptoms and signs.

Cardiovascular disease usually manifests later, but any undue fatigue or shortness of breath on exertion must be investigated. While the annual physical has been found a pretty useless ritual, getting one each decade in your 20s and 30s would seem warranted to listen for heart murmurs, EC/KG abnormalities and lipids. In this age group congenital abnormalities are more to be found than those caused by poor diet.

Infectious and parasitic diseases are usually communicable diseases spread by bacteria or viruses by airborne droplets, insects, and contaminated food; or, they are sexually transmitted. Everyone should be vaccinated against as many illnesses as possible. After that, continue to take care of personal hygiene.

Chronic Respiratory Disease is invariably the result of smoking, either active or passive, tobacco or marijuana and, as such, is preventable. Asthma is also an underestimated chronic illness where research reveals sufferers under-treat themselves. Neglecting regular prevention medication and only seeking immediate emergency relief leads to unnecessary hospitalizations and even deaths. Again, a very preventable illness.

Musculoskeletal Diseases in these statistics don't cause death. They include osteo and rheumatoid arthritis, chronic back pain and even gout, all of which are popularly considered as occurring in the older populace. Back pain increases dramatically at age 20 years (to 54), unlike the arthritides, which increase later at 40 years. There can be no doubt that these conditions can be a severe problem, ever since "man became the only animal with enough arrogance to walk upright on his hind legs." Often a cause cannot be found, and this has led to abuse of the welfare system and a complicated psychiatric roundabout of "pain" gets reward." Much can be prevented by strong core muscles (para-spinal and abdominal), being fit, reducing abdominal fat and avoiding unnatural postures especially while lifting (bend the knees). Back surgery has improved by leaps and bounds.

Nervous System Disorders: At this age these cases are usually epilepsy or multiple sclerosis. Unfortunately, there are no prevention methods except for avoiding traumas that cause epilepsy.

Digestive System Diseases run the spectrum from indigestion to cancer (covered above), and include ulcers, irritable bowel syndrome, Crohn's disease, ulcerative colitis and piles.

Looking ahead, there is a dramatic change after 45, when heart disease and cancer raise their ugly heads. This fact should alert all to cease smoking and eat the ***Newtrition PHYTO Diet (Book 2)***. The most obvious, and therefore frequently the most overlooked deduction, is that heart disease and cancer *don't* suddenly start at 45. If males do manage to live through their high-risk behavior years, avoiding unintentional or intentional injuries, they have, however, *not avoided causing the pathology that will kill or burden them.* So as well as addressing these high-risk behaviors by being alert to possible depression and potential suicide, we should also be looking at what prevents the diseases that manifest after 45.

You will also see that mental illness and suicide dramatically decrease with age. It would be more than cynical to suggest that this is because all the fragile males have already topped themselves. Rather it is the accepted medical wisdom that if we can get them through these high-risk years, their mental state stabilizes to normal, so it's worth being aware and making the effort.

Hearing loss intrudes after 40. Stop exposure to loud noise now.

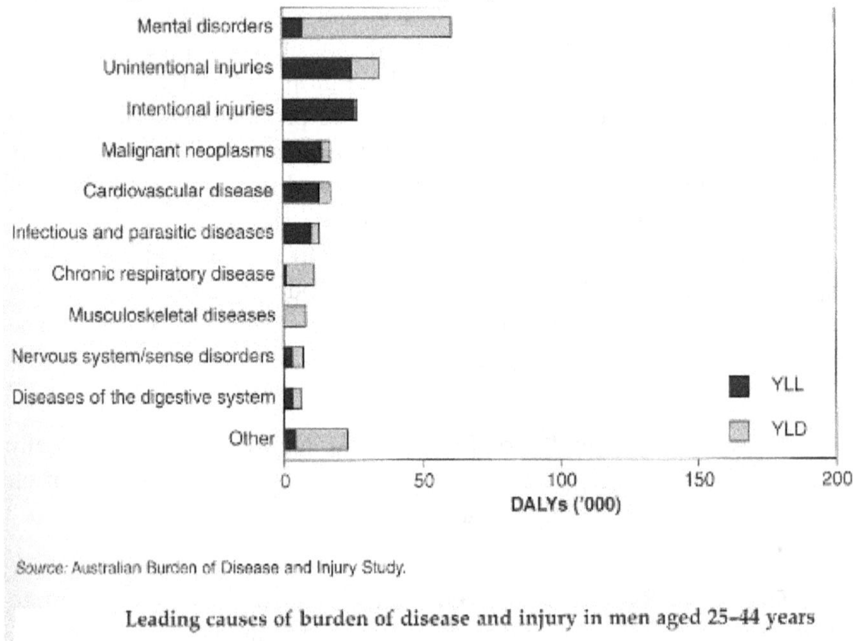

Leading causes of burden of disease and injury in men aged 25–44 years

Light Bar = Premature Disabilities (YLD)
Dark Bar = Premature Deaths (YLL)
DALY = Years lost to both.

17. Men 35–44 -49 UK, 45-64 Australia

" The Male Menopause, Heart Attacks and Cancer"

Overall

The drugs, booze, smoking, junk food, being overweight and unfit have now caught up and cardiovascular disease and cancer affect over half of these men. Look ahead at what illnesses are most likely when over 65. These are what you must now try to prevent, as well as getting early diagnosis of any current ailments (CVD increases significantly at 65 but cancer does not).

Causes of Male Deaths

	USA 35 - 44 years	UK 35 -49	Australia 45-64
1	Suicide	Suicide	CVD
2	Poisoning	Heart Disease	Cancer
3	CAD	Liver Disease	Accidents
4	RTA	Accidental Poisoning	Digestive D
5	Homicide	CVD	Ch Lung D
6	Liver Disease	Lung Cancer	Diabetes melitus
7	Hypertension	RTA	Nervous Syst
8	Diabetes mellitus	CAC	Mental
9	CVA	Lymphoid Cancer	Genito-urinary
10	CAC	Brain Cancer	Musculoskeletal

Causes of Premature Deaths and Disabilities in Order 45-64

1. Cardiovascular disease
2. Malignant neoplasms (cancer)
3. Nervous system disorders
4. Mental disorders (Disability far greater than deaths)
5. Chronic Respiratory Diseases
6. Diabetes mellitus
7. Unintentional injuries
8. Musculoskeletal diseases (100% disabilities)
9. Digestive system diseases
10. Genito-urinary diseases
11. Other

Disabling conditions most affecting 45–64-year-old males:

1. Ischemic heart disease 17%
2. Lung cancer 7%
3. Nervous system 7%
4. Mental disorders 6%
5. COPD (Chronic Obstructive Pulmonary Disease) 5%
6. Diabetes 5%
7. Hearing Loss 5%

Causes of disease and injury burden: Men aged 45–64

1. Cardiovascular disease 26%
2. Ischemic Heart Disease 64%
3. Strokes 17%
4. Cancer 25%
5. Lung 26%
6. Colorectal 16%

What to do:

Get help if depressed or if any suicidal thoughts

At 35 or 40 it is time to get a base-line level for all medical tests as per Section 4: Tests and Diagnoses but especially:

Get BP, lipids, BG, Liver Function Tests and CXR done

Immediately stop smoking

Adopt the Mediterranean Diet of ***Newtrition Foods (Book 2)***

Consider low-dose aspirin twice a week to help prevent stomach

Get fit

Report wheeze, difficult breathing, chronic cough, bloody phlegm

Get a hearing test if any difficulties.

Suicide

It is a surprise that suicide is the number one killer for men aged 35 to 50 years in the USA and England/Wales. One can only conjecture as to the causes, Unfulfilled ambitions, Failed love, Business failure, the Male Menopause but psychiatry for too long has got bogged down as to etiology (cause) and not got on with treatment - rather like asking someone bleeding to death from a leg wound 'how it happened' rather than staunching the loss and applying a tourniquet.

A little known fact is that it is not known how anti-depressants work and that the only reliable anti-depressant over the last 25 years is called Placebo.

All are at risk and the best help is support from all sources, family, health workers, friends, social groups. Any talk of suicide, even a seeming joke, is a red-flag emergency.

Cardiovascular disease

Ischemic Heart Disease means the blood supply to the heart is compromised by cholesterol plaques and narrowing of the coronary (heart) arteries. This usually first manifests as heart pain on exertion (angina) and must be treated and monitored. Any chest pain, undue fatigue or shortness of breath on exertion must be investigated. It would be advisable to get your blood pressure checked, to listen for heart murmurs, and ECG/EKG and lipids (LDL) at ages 35, 45, 55 and 65. Immediately report any transient weakness, loss of movement/coordination or vision.

Cancer

This age group, between 35 and 64, is where cancer is most likely and early diagnosis affords the best chances of cure or survival. Be aware of the early symptoms and signs. Report any cough, loss of weight, altered bowel habit, passing or coughing blood or mucus.

Cancer of the colon (CAC): Unexplained fatigue, loss of weight, change of bowel habit, and passing mucus, slime or blood are symptoms and signs. Get a blood test, and if slightly anemic get a colonoscopy. Fecal blood tests may pick up some, but colonoscopy is the gold standard. People who took an aspirin tablet (325 or 81 mg) at least twice a week (usually for headache or muscle pain) had a lower incidence of gastrointestinal tract cancers, especially colorectal cancers.[76]

USPSTF Recommends Aspirin for Preventing CVD and Colorectal Cancer - But with Reservations

The US Preventive Services Task Force recommends aspirin for primary prevention of cardiovascular disease and colorectal cancer in some high-risk adults in their 50s and 60s. The guidelines, an update of the group's 2007 and 2009 recommendations, are published in the

Annals of Internal Medicine. Low-dose aspirin is recommended for adults aged 50–59 who have at least a 10% risk for a cardiovascular event in the next decade, low bleeding risk, and a life expectancy of at least 10 years; patients must also be willing to take aspirin daily for at least 10 years (grade B recommendation).For people aged 60–69 fitting the above criteria, the decision to start aspirin should be an individual one. For patients younger than 50 and older than 69, there is not enough evidence to make recommendations. Dr. Harlan Krumholz, editor-in-chief of *NEJM Journal Watch Cardiology*, comments: "The recommendations are sensible, but people should realize that they are based on very few high-quality studies—and no recent ones. Ultimately, aspirin's effects are felt to be modest, and the decision [to initiate treatment] is ideal for shared decision-making since there is some uncertainty about the relevance of the evidence to contemporary practice and a trade-off of risks and benefits."

Lung cancer and COPD are invariably due to smoking tobacco or marijuana and are preventable. But be alert to any past workplace contaminants such as asbestos, which may be as "innocent" as lagging on factory or ships' pipes. If you are a smoker you must get regular chest x-rays. If you have a cough that hangs on, also get a chest x-ray. Better still, stop smoking.

Skin Cancer and Melanoma: Like all cancers they "take off" after the age of 40 and increase. This is due to excessive ultraviolet radiation—sun exposure. Like lung cancer it is not the one packet of cigarettes but the regular exposure to the carcinogens (smoke or sun) over some 20 years that initiates the mutation of the DNA in our cells to become cancers. The best feature of skin cancer is that it can be seen and therefore most can be diagnosed early enough to effect a cure. Get checked annually.

Nervous System Disorders: At this age these are multiple sclerosis or more rare degenerative disorders, for which there are no prevention or treatments except for specialized rehab centers. Report any unexplained limb weakness, incoordination, vision disturbances, altered sensations, headaches.

Mental Problems: Usually anxiety or depression. Initially try cognitive behavioral therapy. Get help.

The "Male Menopause" is also a real entity, where the man feels he is losing his youthful vitality and seeks to recreate it with a sports car and trophy mistress. While this may be an object of derision, it has been pointed out that monogamy is unnatural to most species and humans by living much longer have not been "prepared" by evolution for the long monogamous relationships that our new longevity provides. It is a subject too complex to deal with here, but an equitable divorce is better than a poisonous marriage. The ultimate objective being the welfare and prosperity of all concerned.

Asthma and emphysema are also very "underestimated" chronic illnesses where research shows sufferers under-treat themselves, especially as to regular prevention medication rather than immediate emergency relief leading to unnecessary hospitalizations and even deaths. Again, a very preventable illness.

Diabetes 2 we associate with being fat but there are many skinny diabetics. Get a Blood Glucose test.

Musculoskeletal Diseases in these statistics don't cause death. They include osteo and rheumatoid arthritis, chronic back pain and even gout.

Back pain increases dramatically at age 20 years to 54, unlike the arthritides, which increase later at 40 years. There can be no doubt that it can be a severe problem ever since "man became the only animal with enough arrogance to walk upright on his hind legs." Often a cause cannot be found, and this has led to abuse of the welfare system and a complicated psychiatric roundabout of "pain" gets reward." Much can be prevented by strong core muscles (para-spinal and abdominal), being fit, reducing abdominal fat and avoiding unnatural postures especially while lifting. Getting a diagnosis allows for the most appropriate treatment. Physiotherapy, weight loss and having fit muscles, while maintaining flexibility and movement, are all important while using the minimum of analgesics. NSAIDS used as anti-inflammatories, while effective, cause heart attacks and I try to avoid them. There is a pecking order as to cardio toxicity, with Naprosyn being the least toxic.

If it persists a Magnetic Resonance Image (MRI) is mandatory for a diagnosis.

Digestive System Diseases: These run the spectrum from indigestion to cancer (covered above) to ulcers, irritable bowel syndrome, Crohn's Disease, ulcerative colitis and piles. Weight loss and tiredness are often the early symptoms, and the passing of blood or mucus is an early sign.

Genito-urinary: This usually means "prostate trouble," or Benign Prostate Hypertrophy (BPH) where the prostate enlarges, then pushes into the bladder causing frequent urination and nocturia—having to get up at night to void. There are drugs available but one type causes feminizing side effects and reduced libido or performance. An interesting alternative may be one of the erection enhancers—Tadalafil (Cialis)—which in smaller doses relaxes the bladder's small muscle wall and relieves the nocturia. Bladder and kidney cancers are not unknown—report passing any pink-blood urine.

The usual treatment is a TURP - Trans Urethral Resection of the Prostate which is a rather brutal "re-bore' of the penis. Some advanced Radiology Departments offer Prostate Artery Embolization (PAE) with less risk, less pain, and less recovery time than traditional surgery.

Other: For hearing loss, it is most important you become aware as to any reduction in your hearing. While there are different types, most are caused by exposure to loud noise (amplified music, machinery). Reduce exposure. Use earmuffs if using noisy machines. Turn TV and radio down.

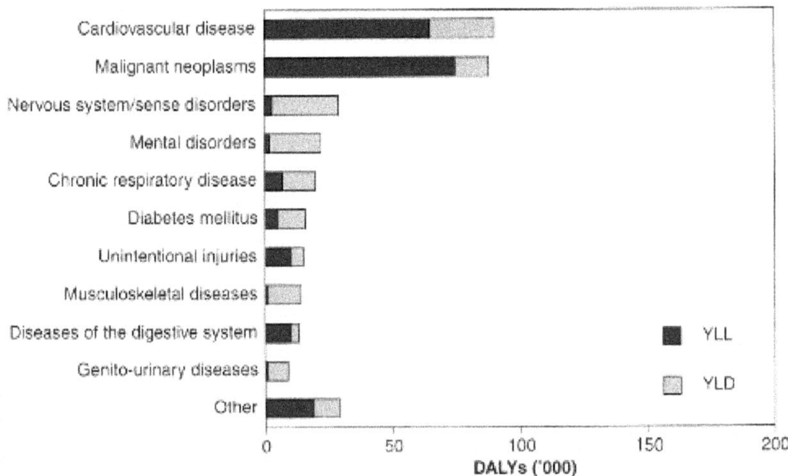

Source: Australian Burden of Disease and Injury Study.

Leading causes of burden of disease and injury in men aged 45–64 years

18. Men 65 years and over

No mental issues: More Fatal Heart Attacks & Cancer

Causes of Deaths and for Australia Disabilities as well

	USA 65 years+	UK 65+	Australia 65+
1	CAD	IHD	CVD
2	Lung Disease	Cancer Lung & Trachea	Cancer
3	Diabetes	Lower Respiratory D	Nervous Syst
4	Stroke	CVD	Ch Lung D
5	Homicide	Ca Prostate	Genito-urinary
6	Cancer Colon		Diabetes melitus
7	Hypertension		Digestive D
8	Cancer Pancreas		Musculoskeletal
9	Liver Cancer		Accidents
10			Endocrine/Metabolic

Thankfully the black Slough of Despond has been crossed and suicide is no longer high on the list.

Both the previous major problems of heart disease and cancer have increased in this age group, and both of these now cause significantly more deaths than disability.

Cardiovascular disease has increased from 26% to 36% (i.e., more than a third), which makes it priority number one. Cancer has only increased by some 2% but it is still one of the major problems.

You are now "old" as seen by those 30 years younger; but as Groucho Mark observed, "You are only as old as the woman you feel," which one observer interpreted as "proving it is never too late to find love."

I am continually amazed at old people who groan as they undress and have to be helped onto the examination table and complain "It's awful getting old, doctor." They are slow, bent, dull and look old, but when I check their age they are up to 10 years younger than I am! Most of them in fact add and admonish me, "Wait till you're my age!" They have no debilitating illnesses but their whole attitude is wrong.

Someone recently said "75 is the new 60"; and due to improved nutrition, public health measures and modern medicine this is indeed the case. So being "65 and over" does not condemn you to the retirement village—rather it is a call to increase your pursuit of health and vitality. Be an optimist. There are a lot of people worse off. When I had whining introspective patients in hospital with not much wrong but who pestered me out of proportion to their ailment, I had them moved beside someone terminally ill; and when that patient died, the change in the hypochondriacs was always startling. One of my "treatments" for bad sleep is to recommend the patient listen to the news. Then after the suicide bombings, refugee drownings, and the ghastly tsunami of bad news upon bad news, the penny drops and they realize they don't have such horrors to contend with. Their anxiety over what was keeping them awake is not as great as these life-and-death struggles; with this new-found objectivity they can go to sleep. But more, this new found objectivity can and should be applied to every-day living. Carpe diem.

We all have to die despite Silicon Valley's efforts, but the whole essence of this book is to live it up as long as you can. Don't become a premature invalid. At 65 and over there is the distinct danger of people winding down because that is how they think society is geared. Well, read *The New York Times* obituaries and see just how many were rock and rollin' into their 90s.

Cardiovascular Disease

Cardiovascular disease is mostly IHD (60%).

Strokes have risen from 17% to 24%.

This is where to place greatest priority. The best advice has been already documented above.

What to do:

Don't smoke

Report any chest pain, shortness of breath, ankle swelling.

Get BP, LDL and BG checked

Get an ECG/EKG to exclude silent atrial fibrillation which is a major cause of strokes and now an epidemic for those over

Learn to feel your own pulse and if thready and irregular, get another ECG/EKG. AF can strike at any time and causes an irregular pulse.

An abdominal ultrasound is now recommended to exclude an aortic aneurysm.

Adopt ***Newtrition PHYTO Diet (Book 2)***, Successful Aging, and Weight programs (lose weight, cope with stress, challenge the brain).

Cancer

Lung cancer accounts for 26%

Prostrate 19%

Colorectal cancer 14%

Skin: get checked annually—more if in a sunbelt area.

What to do:

Get a chest x-ray

Report any urgency, frequency of urination or nocturia (having to get up at nights to void).

Report any alteration of bowel habit, passage of blood, mucus.

There are no satisfactory tests for cancer of the prostate, and in any event it is often so slow growing, men die from something else. It is alleged that every male over 90 has cancer of the prostate.

Consider having a colonoscopy. Cancer of the colon is curable if resected early enough.

Nervous System Disorders

Alzheimer's/Dementia may begin be alert to signs and symptoms (see next sequel books).

See previous section.

It is now more important than ever to accept new challenges and force the brain along and adopt the Newtrition PHYTO Diet.

The Rest

Follow the previous age group. Refer to the above but there is now greater urgency not to ignore what you may consider “minor” symptoms—as can be seen in the patient analysis of "Types" (Section 3) it is the proactive patient who achieves the best results for their health.

Stay fit, slim and active with plenty of new mental challenges.

Finally, see the chapter for age-specific tests and investigations.

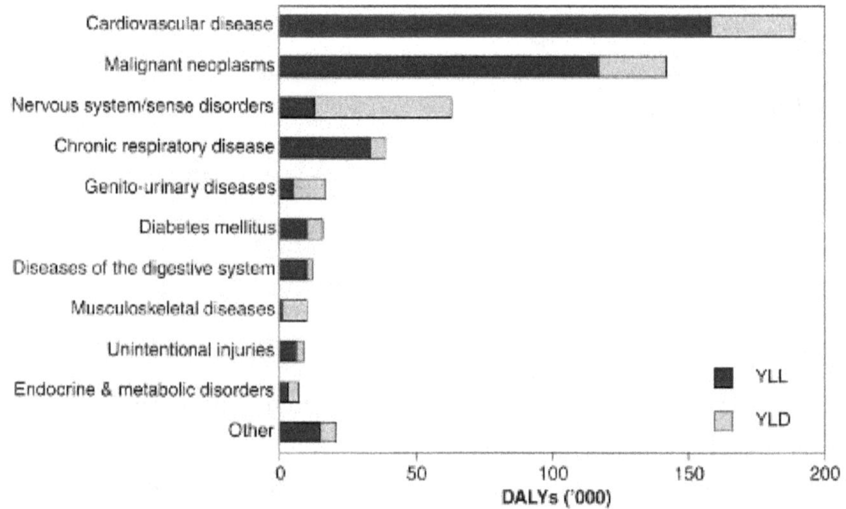

Leading causes of burden of disease and injury in men aged 65 years and over

Light bar = **YLD** = “Healthy” **Years Lost due to Disability** = Non-fatal burden of illness
Dark bar = **YLL** = **Years of Life Lost** due to premature death by the same illness
DALY = YLL + YLD = Total Burden
One DALY is the equivalent of one year of healthy life lost.

19. Women

Overview

Womens' Greatest Concerns (UK)

1. Heart disease
2. Breast cancer
3. Osteoporosis
4. Depression
5. Autoimmune diseases

Leading causes of Burden of Disease and Injury

Condition	% of Total
25 - 44 years	
Depression	12.1
Anxiety	6.2
Breast Cancer	4.9
Genito-urinary Diseases	4.2
Asthma	3.5
45 - 64 years	
Breast Cancer	10.0
Osteoarthritis	6.6
Ischemic Heart Disease	6.5
Diabetes mellitus	5.6
Depression	5.2
65 years and over	
Ischemic Heart Disease	20.3
Stroke	10.7
Alzheimer's / Dementia	8.9
Ch Obstructive Pulmonary Disease	4.0
Breast cancer	3.6

Note: These are conditions which make someone an invalid or disabled and may or may not include the cause of death.

20. Young Women

USA Females 15 - 24	**England and Wales 5 - 19**
RTA	RTA
Suicide	Suicide
Poisonings	Homicide
Homicide	Lymphoid Cancer
Endocrine Disorders	Congenital Defects
Other Injuries	Cerebral palsy
Congenital Anomalies	Brain Cancer
Maternal conditions	Accidental poisoning
Leukemia	Accidental breathing threats
Influenza and Pneumonia	Emphysema / Bronchitis

The England and Wales figures are from age 5 years so more Infantile conditions occur.

For the 15 to 24 years old age group Road Accidents predominate then Suicide and this is where most emphasis needs to be placed.

Counselling not to drink and drive and to wear seat belts cannot be over emphasized or repeated enough.

Suicide watch is all important: Any mood changes, withdrawl, sadness, volatility or frank depression must be given immediate attention and intensive observation and support.

21. Women aged 25–44 years

"Depression, Anxiety and Cancer"

Causes of Female Deaths

	% USA 25 - 34	**ENGLAND & WALES 20-34**	**Australia 25 - 44**
1	Unintentional Injuries 31.2	Poisoning	Suicide
2	Cancer 12.6	Accidental poisoning	Accidental poisoning
3	Suicide 9.3	RTA	RTA
4	Heart Disease 7.4	Breast Ca	CAD

Disabilities

As noted Causes of Premature Death are not always in the same order as Causes of Premature Disabilities.

In this age group Depression and Anxiety far outstrip any cause of deaths where cancer claims most victims. As seen in the following graph extract:

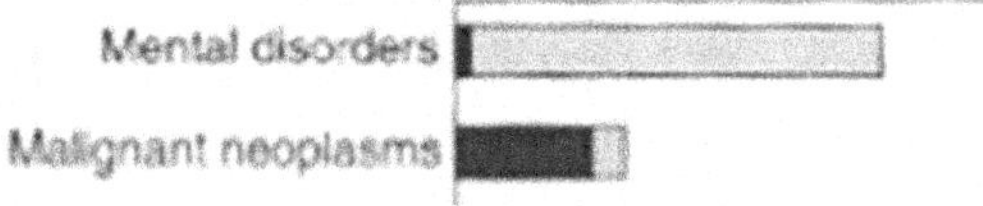

The light bar gives the proportion of Disabilities; the dark bar the amount of deaths. It can easily be seen how non-fatal (light bar) Mental Disorders far outstrip any deaths they may cause whereas the greatest cause of deaths are cancers (Malignant Neoplasms, mostly Breast Cancer) the dark bar below.

Causes of Premature Deaths and Disabilities in Order 25 - 44 yrs

1. Mental disorders (Disability far greater than Deaths)
2. Malignant neoplasms (cancer)
3. Chronic Respiratory Diseases

4. Genito-urinary diseases (100% disability - not fatal)
5. Musculoskeletal diseases (100% disabilities- not fatal)
6. Unintentional injuries
7. Cardiovascular disease
8. Intentional injuries (100% fatal ? connected to 1)
9. Digestive system diseases
10. Nervous system disorders

Disability problems for this age group (25-44 years) are:

1. Mental illnesses

Depression 38%

Anxiety 33%

As a group the greatest cause of disabilities in this 25–44-year-old age group for women is dominated by mental disorders, which in turn are mainly due to depression (38%) and anxiety (33%) causing disability rather than premature deaths.

While deaths, according to this data set, are relatively few, it is to be noted that for "8. Intentional injuries", by which we can only assume suicide, deaths are 100% and surely the result of a mental illness be it acute or chronic depression. (In one of the later Live Longest Books I discuss Depression as being "Reactive" or "Endogenous" where basically some shattering broken romance may cause an acute depression and suicide as distinct from some slipping into the "black abyss" when there is no apparent reason. But while ostensibly "relatively few they are absolutely devastating to the survivors and the families, and all such patients must be watched like hawks.

Drugs or illicit substances do not seem to play as much a role as with young men, but the liberation of women may make this an impression rather than an actual fact. After all, women are smoking and drinking alcohol more, which usually shadows drug and substance abuse.

The explosion of hormones provides a roller coaster ride for many young women with unrealized and confused ambitions. Marrying your childhood sweetheart and having kids before the age of 20 is no longer the preferred career move. But what is? A world perceived to be male-dominated and offering less career satisfaction might frustrate, confuse and depress the more ambitious. Coping with the workplace and accepting responsibility can engender anxiety in those promoted beyond their experience or competence. A turbulent home life only exacerbates the problem(s).

Most seem to settle in their 30s but the "Big 4-0" would seem to make women sit up, look around and wonder if there isn't more to life and wonder if it isn't passing them by.

While unpleasant, most of these mental disorders respond to treatment and do not account for many deaths.

Cancer

Cancer accounts for 13% of the disabilities in this age group, of which breast cancer predominates at 37% and is the one of the greatest causes of death. Early diagnosis is essential.

What to do:

Mammograms, examinations and pap smears should be done.

Genetic counseling if there is a family history.

Chronic Respiratory Disease

This is essentially the same as the advice for men (above).

Genito-Urinary Disease

Sexually Transmitted Diseases (STD) are likely and increasing in the sexually active with multiple partners. Intercourse, childbirth and the anatomy where the opening of the urethra is so close to the vagina and anus make women much more susceptible to urinary tract infections. It is essential that these be completely cleared each time or there is the chance of chronic infection, which can then ascend to the kidney—a far greater problem. The gold standard is to get a mid-stream urine specimen to identify the germ, and the best antibiotic, and then repeat it after the course to make sure the urine is now sterile.

Childbirth can also distort the anatomy, making infections more easily acquired as well as causing the uterus to displace.

Regular checks and pap smears are mandatory.

Musculoskeletal

Musculoskeletal disorders don't often cause death and include osteo and rheumatoid arthritis and chronic back pain. Back pain increases dramatically at age 20 years to 54, unlike the arthritides, which increase later at 40 years. There can be no doubt that it can be a severe problem. Often a cause cannot be found. Much can be prevented by strong core muscles (para-spinal and abdominal), being fit, reducing abdominal fat and avoiding unnatural postures especially while lifting. Getting a diagnosis allows for the most appropriate treatment. Physiotherapy, weight loss and having fit muscles, while maintaining flexibility and movement, all are important, while using the minimum of analgesics. NSAIDS used as anti-inflammatories, while effective, cause heart attacks and I try to avoid them. There is a pecking order as to cardio toxicity, with naproxen being the least toxic.

Cardiovascular Disease (CVD)

CVD surprisingly manifests later in women or is under-diagnosed. Any undue fatigue, shortness of breath on exertion or chest pain must be investigated. Get BP checked regularly and an ECG/EKG if asymptomatic when you hit 40, your LDL at 30, as a baseline record.

Digestive Tract Disorders

Digestive system diseases run the spectrum from indigestion and cancer (covered above) to ulcers, irritable bowel syndrome, Crohn's Disease, ulcerative colitis and piles. Weight loss and tiredness are often the early symptoms, while the passing of blood or mucus is an early sign. Recurrent abdominal pain, swelling or diarrhea must be investigated.

Nervous System Disorders

At this age these are Multiple Sclerosis or rare degenerative disorders for which there are no prevention or treatments except for specialized rehab centers.

The following Graphs are to show the proportions as to different Causes of Premature Deaths (UK) and then the most helpful combining Causes of both Premature Deaths and Disabilities.

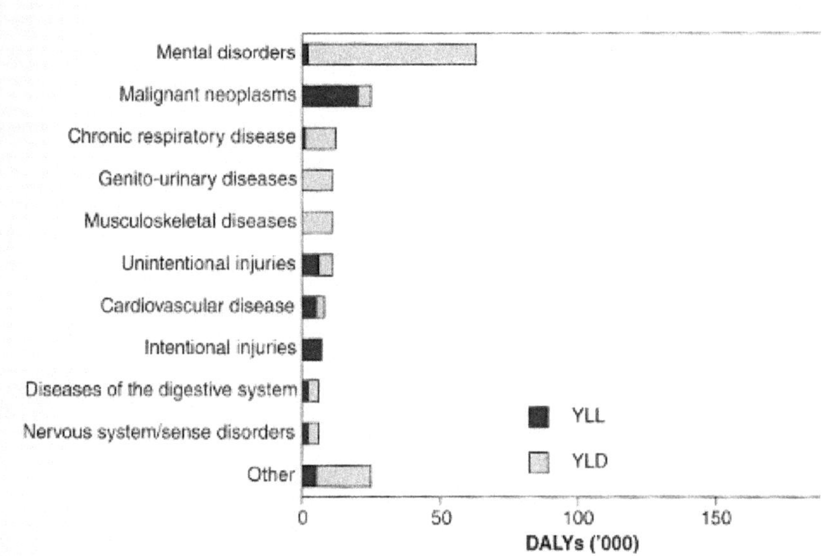

Source: Australian Burden of Disease and Injury Study.

Leading causes of burden of disease and injury in women aged 25–44 years

Light Bar = Premature Disabilitiy

Dark Bar = Premature Deaths

22. Women Aged 45–64 Years

"Cancer (breast, lung, colon) and Heart "

Causes of Premature Deaths

	% USA 45 - 54	ENGLAND & WALES 35-49	Australia 45 -64
1	Cancer (Breast, Lung, CRC) 32.8	Breast Ca	CAD
2	Heart Disease 15.1	Liver D	Lung Ca
3	Unintentional injuries 9.7	Accidental poisoning	Breast Ca
4	Ch Liver D 4.2	Suicide	Suicide
5	Ch Lower Respiratory D 3.5	IHD	CRC

Australia Causes of Premature Deaths and Disabilities

1. Malignant neoplasms (cancer) 13%
2. Cardiovascular disease 5.7%
3. Mental disorders (Disability far greater than deaths)
4. Musculoskeletal diseases (100% disabilities- not fatal)
5. Nervous system disorders
6. Chronic Respiratory Diseases
7. Diabetes mellitus
8. Unintentional injuries
9. Digestive system diseases
10. Oral health

This is quite a difference from the younger previous group wherein the dominant mental issues of Depression and Anxiety and Intentional injuries have been displaced by Cancer and Heart Disease and surprisingly no Genito-urinary issues - presumably addressed in the earlier sexually active and child-bearing age group. The Respiratory diseases are mostly due to smoking then asthma but Diabetes mellitus (Type 1 - insulin dependent) makes its first appearance while oral health makes its first and only appearance. Time to get your teeth fixed - pity about the lack of fluoride as a kid.

Problems for age 45–64 women:

This is the most dangerous age for breast cancer, but other cancers occur as well, while heart disease and strokes impact.

Cancer

Breast cancer 30%

Lung 14%

Colorectal 13%.

Cardiovascular Disease 14%

IHD 47%

Strokes 29%

Mental Disorders

Depression 51%.

Anxiety 33%

Osteoarthritis 7%

Diabetes 6%

The cancer and cardiovascular disease are more often fatal, whereas the others more often result in non-fatal burdens.

Menopause

Varies from mild to severe. Not much helps except Hormone Replacement Therapy (HRT) which has received bad reports but these have been found to not be as bad as originally thought.

What to do:

Breast Cancer

1 in 8 women will develop cancer of the breast.

Regular examinations by your doctor.

Learn to self-examine—you have more time than anyone else.

Regular mammograms. Mammograms are arguably the best screen test, but some 1 in 6 cancers are missed.

Have regular pap smears.

Lung Cancer

Don't smoke

Get a chest x-ray or CT scan / MRI if coughing blood / losing weight

Lung cancer and COPD are invariably due to smoking tobacco or marijuana and are preventable. But be alert to any past workplace contaminants such as asbestos, which may be as "innocent" as lagging on factory or ships' pipes or on old roofs and walls.

Colorectal Cancer

Have a colonoscopy if any passage of blood or mucus.

Cardiovascular Disease

Ischemic heart disease means the blood supply to the heart is compromised by cholesterol plaques and narrowing of the coronary (heart) arteries This usually first manifests as heart pain on exertion (angina) and must be treated and monitored.

Report any chest pain or heat flutters—possible ECG/EKG

Also see note regarding aspirin in relevant men's' age group.

Strokes

Make sure you are on a low-dose pill.

Skin Cancer and Melanoma

Like all cancers they "take off" after the age of 40 and increase. This is due to excessive ultraviolet radiation—sun exposure. Like lung cancer it is not the one packet of cigarettes but the regular exposure to the carcinogens (smoke or sun) over some 20 years that initiates the mutation of the DNA in our cells to become cancers. The best feature of skin cancer is that it can be seen, and therefore most can be diagnosed early enough to effect a cure. Get checked annually.

Mental Issues

Treat depression / anxiety – Cognitive Behavioral Therapy maybe preferable to drugs.

By now suicide seems to not be the potential threat it is with younger women, so support is what is needed.

The average age for menopause is 53 and this comes as a psychological as well as hormonal insult. It is only the human, the pilot whale and one other animal which undergoes menopause. Here the estrogen is abruptly cut off. It is a violent hormonal change with no male equivalent but obviously can herald many mixed emotions.

Osteo Arthritis

My best analogy is that OA is "rust" in the joints. It can run the gamut from inconsequential to being completely debilitating.

Report any finger joint lumps, and hand, knee, or hip pain or stiffness.

Keeping mobile (like moving and using a rusty hinge) is all-important.

Diabetes

Get a Random Blood Glucose test.

As noted elsewhere, diabetes 2 is usually associated with being overweight, but I have some very slim and fit diabetics in my practice, and some with no family history.

The first line of treatment is to adopt the ***Newtrition PHYTO Diet (Book 2)***.

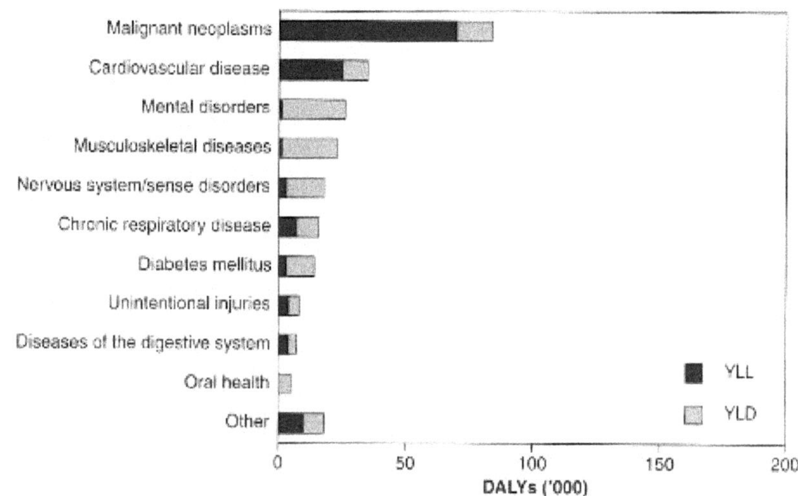

Source: Australian Burden of Disease and Injury Study.

Leading causes of burden of disease and injury in women aged 45-64 years

---

Dark band = Premature Deaths

Light band = Premature Disabilities

23. Women 65 years and over

"Oh my (irregularly) Beating Heart "

% USA 65 - 74	ENGLAND & WALES 65-79	Australia 65 - 74
Cancer 35.1	Lung and Trachea Ca	Lung Ca
Heart Disease 18.1	Ch Lower Respiratory D	CAD
Ch Lower Respiratory D 8.6	IHD	COPD
Stroke 4.5	Dementia & Alzheimer's	CVD
Diabetes 3.7	CVD	CRC

Cardiovascular problems now take over from cancer as the greatest cause of disabilities.

The early signs of Dementia and Alzheimer's manifest; eyesight and hearing start to deteriorate.

Heart attacks and strokes present most problems: Control of Blood Pressure and any heart arrhythmias must be checked and controlled.

Mental disorders have disappeared and teeth have been fixed.

Eyesight and hearing problems manifest.

The early signs of Dementia and Alzheimer's manifest and Nervous System disorders, rare in the younger such as Parkinson's Disease manifest with increasingly small handwriting, frozen expression, shuffling and "pill rolling" tremors suggesting Parkinson's.

As noted in the men's section but repeated here, you are now "old," but as with the age-old saying, "You are only as old as you feel"; in other words, you can still have "joie de vivre"—the joy of life.

I am continually amazed at these old people who groan as they undress and have to be helped onto the examination table and complain "It's awful getting old, doctor." They are slow, bent, dull and look old, but when I check their age they are up to 10 years younger than I am! Most of them in fact add and admonish me, "Wait till you're my age"!? They have no debilitating illnesses but their whole attitude is wrong.

Someone recently said, "75 is the new 65"; and due to improved nutrition, public health measures and modern medicine this is indeed the case. So being "65 and over" does not condemn you to the retirement village but rather is a call to increase your pursuit of health and vitality. Be an optimist. There are a lot of people worse off. When I had whining introspective patients in hospital with not much wrong but who pestered me out of proportion to their ailment, I had them moved close to someone terminally ill and when that patient died, the change in the hypochondriacs was always startling. One of my "treatments" for bad sleep is to recommend the patient listen to the news. After the suicide bombings, refugee drownings, and the ghastly tsunami of bad news on bad news, the penny drops and they don't have such horrors to contend with. Their anxiety over what was keeping them awake is not as great as these misfortunes; they realize some objectivity and they go to sleep.

We all have to die, but the whole essence of this book is to live it up and stay healthy as long as you can. Don't become a premature invalid or prematurely old because of a bad mental attitude. At 65 and over there is the distinct danger of people winding down because that is how they think society is geared. Well, read *The New York Times* obituaries and see just how many were rock and rollin' into their 90s.

The main health problems in older women are:

Cardiovascular 37.2%

IHD is the main cardiovascular problem at 54.4%, then stroke at 28.8%.

Cancer 20.8%

Colorectal cancer 16.4%

Breast 15.1%

Lung 15.1%.

Nervous system disorders 17.9%

Of which Alzheimer's / dementia 49.7%

Hearing and vision loss 32.1%

Parkinson's 12.2%

Acute Respiratory Infections

What to do:

An ECG/EKG is now mandatory to rule out silent atrial fibrillation and reduce strokes.

Colon cancer has now overtaken breast cancer, so report any change of bowel habit, undue/unexplained fatigue or anemia, and chronic diarrhea; consider a colonoscopy.

Continue mammograms and breast examinations.

Report any ongoing coughs.

Get a chest x-ray if there is past history of smoking.

Staying fit with mental challenges is all-important. Alzheimer's and Parkinson's, while inevitable, can be remarkably delayed by doing so. Even ballroom dancing and bridge helps.

Get eyes and hearing checked.

Report any tremors, shuffling, smaller writing.

Get any chest infections treated aggressively and promptly. Review and do annually.

Get skin checked more regularly if damaged and living in a sunbelt zone.

Many of these deaths and disabilities may seem sudden, like a heart attack or a stroke; but in truth, most have been brewing and incubating for decades. If we are at our healthiest at age 11, then by 40 years our tests reveal a sudden spurt of bad results. Most of these we don't notice. Our raised blood pressure and blood lipids are asymptomatic; we may be a little more thirsty and void more from diabetes, but the joint pains are usually mild and just starting, and any symptoms of cancer are not usually flagrant—perhaps a little tiredness, usually passed off. And so, most usually from self-inflicted abuse of high-risk behaviors, we have spent three decades, from 10 to 40 years of age, accumulating damage. The only outside signs are overweight/obesity and the only one we notice is pushing the paper farther away to read.

Perhaps life doesn't begin at 40.

Causes of Premature Deaths and Disabilities in Order

1. Cardiovascular disease
2. Malignant neoplasms (cancer)
3. Nervous system disorders
4. Chronic Respiratory Diseases
5. Musculoskeletal diseases (100% disabilities- not fatal)
6. Diabetes mellitus
7. Digestive system diseases
8. Unintentional injuries
9. Genito-urinary diseases
10. Acute Respiratory diseases

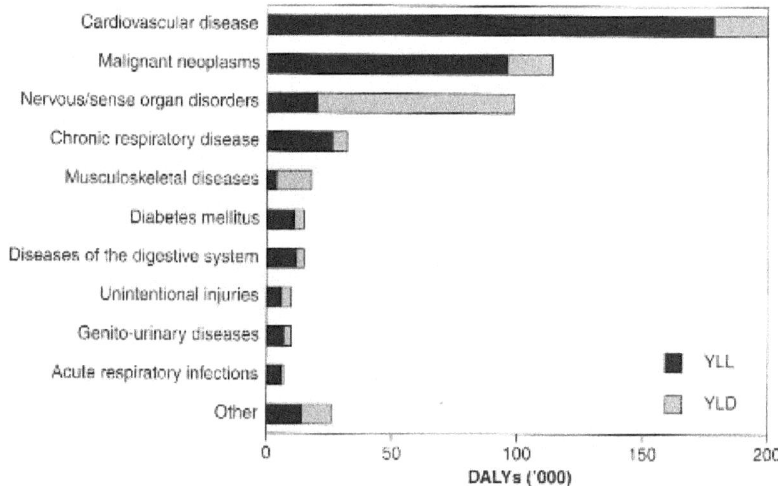

Source: Australian Burden of Disease and Injury Study.

Leading causes of burden of disease and injury in women aged 65 years and over

Light bar = **YLD** = "Healthy" **Years Lost due to Disability** = Non-fatal burden of illness
Dark bar = YLL = Years of Life Lost due to premature death by the same illness
DALY = YLL + YLD = Total Burden
One DALY is the equivalent of one year of healthy life lost.

24. Overall Male and Female

When young high risk and even low risk (but cumulative) behaviors are often treated as a "rite of passage' or relegated to be addressed when older. Drinking and now binge drinking are epidemic. Smoking has gratifyingly been recognized as 'not cool' but a stupid, injurious affectation and drug of addiction.

Cars pull up beside me with speakers that would do Carnegie Hall justice with some young man with a baseball cap on backwards gyrating to the beat, which seems to lift his car off the ground but ensuring his accelerated hearing loss. Meanwhile in my rear-vision mirror some 18 year old or so girl is tailgating me until she cuts me off with the one-finger salute and absolutely no idea how to control a skid. And both of these are drinking a Cola and eating pizza or some processed food and are overweight. The only exercise they get is their thumbs texting on their Smart-Phones. They have little or no idea of nutrition or hygiene and getting a tan is most desirable.

While Sir William Osler observed how humans have a great desire to take pills, as a doctor there is simply no-way I could ever take something made by some criminal without any quality control or guaranteed dose. That is simply crazy - suicidal in fact.

I have no answer to these behaviors other than alerting those readers under 40 years of age, or their parents or anyone (!) to these avoidable disorders let alone fatal illnesses.

Of course, I was perfect and never indulged in such practices...Pig's Bottom...I often say the only reason I'm alive is that when I arrived at the Pearly Gates (or was it the other place) the "Use By Date" on my forehead was blurred and they sent me back.

But a friend of mine, a Rock 'N Roll Drummer, who, of course has a hearing loss, told me how he "wished someone had told him to wear ear-plugs and the dangers of loud noise". But I don't think he would have listened - (bad pun).

But hopefully a word in a not yet hearing-impaired ear at least may alert and prevent this avoidable damage.

The Earlier You Start, the Less Downstream Problems

For preventing early deaths the following high-risk behaviors must be addressed:

Tobacco – cigarette smoking

Processed foods

Eating habits – processed and junk foods – lack of fruit/vegetables

Exercise patterns – physical inactivity

High blood pressure

Drinking habits – alcohol harm

Weight – overweight/underweight

High LDL

Driving style

Hobbies – high risk - head trauma from sport

Occupations – high risk

Pesticides, industrial-workplace toxins (nail salons)

Diesel fumes / Air pollution

Unsafe sex

Illicit drugs

Lack of vaccinations

Hygiene

Loud music, noise

Glare

Sunburn

Overall (all age) Non-Fatal Burdens of Diseases

1. IHD (Ischemic Hearty Disease) 12
2. Stroke 5
3. COPD (Chronic Obstructive Pulmonary (Lung) Disease) 4
4. Depression 4
5. Lung cancer 4
6. Prescription Drugs (never listed a causing death or disability)
7. Dementia 3.5
8. Diabetes 3
9. Colon Cancer 3
10. Asthma 2.5
11 Osteoarthritis 2.2
12 Suicide 2.2
13 MVA 2.2 Motor Vehicle Accident)
14 Breast Cancer 2.2

Overall Prevention: What to Control. The Treatment, Not Error, Is Biggest Risk to Elderly

The greatest threat to older patients' safety in primary care is the risk posed by treatment itself, not treatment error or negligence, according to an analysis of no-fault claims data from New Zealand. Medication injuries were the main source (34%) of all treatment injuries among the elderly, and within that category, antibiotics were, by far, the biggest culprit (51%). Next highest among injury sources were nonsteroidal anti-inflammatory drugs (9%) and angiotensin-converting enzyme inhibitors (9%). Antibiotics also topped the list for causes of serious or sentinel injuries for patients aged 65 years and older. Antibiotics caused 39% of such injuries in that age group, followed by warfarin (14%) and steroids (7%). The serious/sentinel category was defined as having "the potential to result in" or "has resulted in" "unanticipated death or major permanent loss of function." Most medication injuries overall were allergic and idiosyncratic reactions, without a suggestion of error (1295; 91% of medication injuries and 34% of all injuries), according to the study. The elderly are particularly susceptible to antibiotic injury, the author notes, because they often are taking multiple medications, leaving them vulnerable to drug–drug interactions. Even when medications can be reconciled, it does not take into account everything a patient is taking over the counter.[77]

More Elderly Using Dangerous Drug Combinations

One in six older adults now regularly use potentially deadly combinations of prescription and over-the-counter medications and dietary supplements—a twofold increase over a 5-year period. While it is not known how many older adults in the United States die of drug interactions, the risk seems to be growing, and public awareness is lacking.

25. What's Up, Doc?

These statistics vary slightly from country to country and year to year but they show how patients' immediate concerns are different from long-term conditions, causes of death and disabilities. The danger is that, by going to the doctor only when we are sick, we ignore the bigger health problems that prematurely kill or disable us as they are asymptomatic.

Prevalent Health Problems: Why We Go To The Doctor (%)

1. Dental caries --
2. Hearing loss 16
3. Endentulism (loss of teeth) 7.6
4. Asthma 6.6
5. Periodontal D 5.6
6. Iron anemia 4
7. Alcohol abuse 4
8. Osteoarthritis 3
9. Chronic Back pain 3.2
10. Depression 3
11. Diabetes 2 2.6
12. Slipped disc 1.9
13. Incontinent urine 1.7
14. Chronic Obstructive Pulmonary Disease (COPD) 1.6
15. Social phobia 1.6
16. Anxiety disorder 1.6
17. Burns/scalds 1.3
18. Benign Prostatic Hypertrophy 1.1
19. Peptic ulcer 1.0
20. Attention Deficit D (ADD) 0.9
21. Cannabis abuse 0.9
22. Cataracts 0.9
23. Angina 0.9
24. Osteoporosis 0.8
25. Bipolar Disorder 0.7

Reasons For Attending The Doctor per 1000 patients

1. URTIs 2370 (Upper Respiratory Tract Infections)
2. Dental Caries 594
3. Chronic. Back pain 330
4. Diarrhea 205
5. LRTIs 190 (Lower Respiratory Tract Infections)
6. Otitis media 56
7. Periodontal Disease 22
8. Depression 21
9. Falls 20
10. Skin cancers 15
11. Alcohol abuse 9
12. Peptic ulcer 9
13. Slipped disc 8
14. Hearing loss 6
15. Menstrual problems 6
16. Motor Vehicle Accident (MVA) 5
17. Diverticulitis 4
18. Anxiety disorder 4
19. Sports injuries 4
20. Asthma 4
21. Gall bladder Disease 4
22. Stroke 3
23. Prostate hypertrophy 3
24. Interpersonal violence 3
25. Angina

Reasons Attending The Doctor (%) one decade later

1. Check-up 9
2. Prescription 7.1
3. Cough 4.5
4. Test results 3.6
5. Vaccination 3.1
6. Sore throat 2.5
7. Back complaint 2.3
8. Rash 1.9
9. Fever 1.5
10. URTI 1.4
11. Headache 1.4
12. Abdominal pain 1.3
13. Depression 1.3
14. Hypertension 1.2
15. Nasal problem 1.2
16. Ear pain 1.1
17. Diarrhea 1.0
18. Tiredness 1.0
19. Administrative 1.0
20. Knee complaint 0.9

Most Managed Problems By The Doctor (%)

1. Hypertension 6.1
2. URTI 4.4
3. Vaccination 3.2
4. Depression 2.4
5. Lipid disorder 2.1
6. Diabetes 2.0
7. Back pain 1.8
8. Bronchitis 1.8
9. Osteoarthritis 1.8
10. Prescription 1.4
11. Check-up 1.3
12. Esophageal Disease 1.3
13. Female genital/pap 1.2
14. Sprain 1.2
15. Urinary Tract Infection 1.2
16. Sleep problems 1.1
17. Anxiety 1.1
18. Menopausal symptoms 1.0

Most Commonly Reported Long-Term Conditions

CONDITION	MALE %	FEMALE %	TOTAL %
Long-sightedness	20.4	24.3	22.4
Short-sightedness	18.3	23.5	20.9
Back pain / disc disorders	21.0	20.7	20.9
Hay fever / allergic rhinitis	15.1	15.9	15.6
Arthritis (all forms)	11.7	15.8	13.9
Asthma	10.5	12.6	11.6
Chronic sinusitis	8.9	12.4	10.5
Deafness (total/partial)	14.2	7.7	10.8
Hypertension	9.7	10.7	10.3
Presbyopia	9.1	9.0	9.0
Migraine	3.6	8.7	6.2
CONDITION	**MALE %**	**FEMALE %**	**TOTAL %**
High cholesterol	6.5	5.6	6.1
Astigmatism	3.9	5.3	4.6
Anxiety disorders	3.4	5.6	4.5
Mood disorders	3.4	5.5	4.5
Bronchitis/emphysema	3.5	3.6	3.6
Diabetes (all forms)	3.0	2.9	3.0
GIT ulcers	2.8	2.7	2.7
Varicose veins	1.1	3.5	2.3
Hernia	2.5	1.6	2.0
Cataract	1.5	2.4	2.0
Tachycardia	1.7	2.1	1.9
Psoriasis	1.5	2.0	1.8
Neoplasms/cancers	2.0	1.4	1.7
Osteoporosis	0.6	2.5	1.6
Edema	1.0	2.1	1.6
Angina	1.6	1.2	1.4
Rheumatism	1.3	1.4	1.3

Anemias	0.3	2.3	1.3
Hemorrhoids	1.0	1.2	1.1
Dermatitis/eczema	1.0	1.2	1.1

Source: Aihw Analysis Of Abs 2001 National Health Survey.

The immediate attention and treatment of even minor illnesses leads to better overall and long-term health. And so, knowing what "minor" illnesses are going around and what new illnesses seem to be evolving, as above, should persuade you to *"get it seen, get it diagnosed and get it better."*

Vomiting and diarrhea, severe chest or abdominal pain, cuts, bleeding, possible fractures, fits, loss of consciousness and acute dramatic episodes... any of these will alarm us and propel us to the doctor post-haste; but the laying down of cholesterol plaque in our coronary arteries, our greatest cause of death by a long shot, is painless and unrealized. This insidious non-acute slow deterioration of our bodies slithers along insidiously, without any dramatic symptoms to alert us.

And so the acute illnesses and the sub-clinical, chronic degeneration go on together; but both must be "seen, diagnosed and fixed." When there are no symptoms or signs, however, it is practically impossible for a layperson to identify, let alone "treat." Prevention, however, is better than treatment.

If we are to live as long as we should, these acute urgent illnesses must be seen, diagnosed and fixed (see chapter 18); as these allegedly "minor" conditions can have profound later downstream effects on our overall health. Who would have thought "hearing loss" was the second most prevalent illness? Perhaps when we or our children are attending a rock concert, turning up the boom box, jamming the earphones in and turning up the volume, we might try and arrange a conversation with an old hearing-impaired (deaf) person. What people with good hearing fail to realize is just how socially isolating deafness can be. These people exist in a silent world and cannot enjoy usual social events—parties, movies, let alone a chat. And such social isolation leads to a shorter lifespan.

Hearing loss is also costly, even in middle-aged individuals: individuals with a diagnosis of hearing loss had 33% higher health care payments compared to patients without hearing loss. Age-related hearing loss affects more than 60% of US adults older than 70 years; the onset is gradual, with prevalence tripling from the age of 50 years to 60 years; but early, successful intervention may prevent future hearing-related disabilities and decreased quality of life. This finding indicates that negative health-related effects of hearing loss, a condition that many consider simply an unavoidable result of aging, may manifest earlier than is generally recognized and may affect use of health care across the continuum of care.[80]

Wearing earplugs during a loud music concert might help prevent hearing loss. Of 50 adults attending an outdoor music festival for 4.5 hours, roughly 8% of the earplug users had a temporary threshold shift on audiogram, indicating hearing loss, compared with 42% in the unprotected group. After the festival, reported rates of new tinnitus were higher in the unprotected group (40% vs. 12%). It was recommended that earplug use "should be actively promoted and encouraged" to help prevent noise-induced hearing loss.[81]

And who among us knew holes in teeth were the most prevalent health condition? The Loonies, Luddites and Leftovers rave against fluoride as they sail off the edge of their Flat Earth while not vaccinating their children. While polio can kill or lead to immediate limb paralysis, having rotten teeth is not as dramatic but it can lead to heart disease, poor nutrition and a shorter life in the long term.

The statistics on disabilities and death don't list alcohol abuse, but it is the seventh most prevalent condition; and many acts of violence, causing death, are the direct result, as well as work accidents and absenteeism. Unless controlled, it is a long-term time bomb. Ice and Crystal Meth are rapidly taking over—especially in remote and rural areas.

Turning the handles of frying pans and saucepans into the wall prevents burns and scalds. Acute sunburn is a documented contributor to melanoma and skin cancers. People who live in sunbelt areas have more cataracts. Sunglasses are mandatory, even on kids, and don't leave them on the desk when you go to lunch.

Depression is being more widely recognized and treated—perhaps even over-diagnosed and over-treated. Try cognitive behavior therapy.

Other conditions listed usually warrant investigation also: slipped disc, low back pain, asthma, urinary symptoms and angina (too often brushed off as "indigestion"). Any chest pain lasting more than 30–40 minutes warrants investigating.

While some of these acute reasons for visiting the doctor may seem trivial, as pointed out with respect to deafness, the long-term effects are profound and lead to a shorter lifespan. Thus my advice: "Get it seen; get it diagnosed; get it fixed."

It is interesting how eyesight accounts for the greatest proportion of conditions in the top 20. Therefore it should not be such a surprise that increased longevity and reduced disabilities are significantly improved by cheaper, more available and quicker cataract surgery.[82]

Most of us would not think, especially when we are young, that reduced vision would or could be a major cause of premature death or disabilities. But reduced vision is a daily impost to Quality of Life (QOL) and therefore is often a preventable cause of premature death or disability. In a different way, increasing deafness also imposes a daily handicap, culminating in increasing social isolation and again reduced QOL and premature death or disabilities.

Conclusions

Thirty of these conditions can be prevented or treated and many are curable if caught early enough. Many more illnesses than we think are preventable. Now we must learn how.

Initial neglect can see many of these acute, curable illnesses become long-term problems.

Now we know what we are in for, how can we prevent them and optimize our health? Before we address the specific programs in the next chapters, there is an overall approach, with advice according to which personality type of patient gets the best results. Then, the easiest analogy to understand preventive medicine is a comparison to how we look after our cars: "Preventive Maintenance."

While compression of morbidity may not be working, in the United States it is because the socioeconomic classes four and five continue to eat rubbish and avoid good medical advice. If you read the chapter on this topic, you will learn to avoid nursing homes and be staggered as to who is making money from "health."

Preventive medicine is simply not practiced much or well. Patients do not want to pay for advice. They Google the latest fad diet and think they know more than the doctor—and maybe they do, since the doctor is too busy with the acute or hospital cases, and preventive medicine has become a backwater.

Finally, some information from trials and studies is offered. Researchers are desperate for funding and so they publish dubious articles and make inflated claims—how do you know where the truth lies? Even the best medical journals have been fooled. Often lurking behind these trials are the drug companies making millions if not billions, suppressing any bad results until many deaths are exposed before they come clean and withdraw their product. Be careful.

Section 3:

What To Do

"What is the most expensive bed in the world? A hospital bed."

26. Gentility

My father taught me "gentility is the best anesthetic." This advice covered everything from injections to treating patients in toto; from handling of tissues during operations, to examining their limbs, to adroitly calming their fears during consultations and problems. Gentility informs my basic recommendations on lifestyle, diet, exercise, aging, care and treatments. For me it has proven to be true, endlessly and every day. It costs no more, but above all, it achieves a better result. I am not talking about being sickly-sweet, simpering, with limp hand-wringing, or about "toxic parenting," which is terrifying in itself—but the calm, reassuring, soft but firm touch, and often a joke to distract them.

Toxic parenting or partnering is defined as "all care and no responsibility." It manifests where the parent(s) or partner are forever expressing their profound concern for their child or relative... but do very little or nothing about fixing any problem. They are like people at an accident who scream out, "Get an ambulance" but don't do it themselves, let alone go and help the victims. I do not think gushing over a patient helps them unless and until a diagnosis and actual help has been provided. It was my job at one hospital to go around fixing up the mistakes of the "nice" doctors who got the chocolates at Christmas from the patients they nearly killed. Gentility need not be gushing; calm reassurance can be one of the gentlest of acts.

While I boast about "being healthy," I have nevertheless suffered quite an amount of significant injuries, all of which were mostly self-inflicted sports injuries due to a congenital defect in my overestimating my own prowess (or underestimating the opposition). But I recovered from them all to still function well enough to work and operate some 10 hours a day at the age of 75 and now 76. I recovered from my injuries by what I call "progressive gentility," which I feel proves this approach and which I emphasize. It was rammed into us medical students by a rather stupid professor of anatomy (he was so incompetent, despite graduating in medicine, he was never registered to practice) who nevertheless taught that "function determines design." In this he was not stupid and it is the only thing for which I am grateful to him.

As a practical example, if you had a broken arm then, when mended, you should *gently* force it to perform those actions you need to do—rather than cosset it to become fixed and limited. I am not advising pushing it through the pain barrier but rather up to the pain barrier (nature's way of telling you something)—and doing it regularly such that you can do a little more each day or week, until its full function is restored as much as possible. This way the broken bones redesign themselves to accommodate the function required.

I once ran one of the first sports clinics (there were not too many around in 1968), where the worst patients were the elite and international sportsmen. Most wouldn't let their injuries heal and went back too soon or had some strange beliefs and systems. And so it is with most people in their ordinary day-to-day lives—wanting it immediately and adopting hair-brained fads. My approach is different: the gentle but progressive resumption to normal function and health. As a very experienced glider pilot friend always counseled me: "No violent movements of the controls."

I have also documented good and legitimate studies, but there are many confusing contradictions. Do we not eat fat? Do we exercise to exhaustion? The answers are a cautious, if not a resounding, "No"! We can eat fat; exercising to exhaustion has more against than for it.

The food faddists insisted we should not eat fat or eggs or salt or whatever... but more careful analysis has found there was no evidence as to fat, and that sugar may be worse than salt. Way back in the 1950s the Mediterranean Diet was a breakthrough whose benefits keep being proven today. My **"Live Longest Newtrition" PHYTO Diet"** foods are unashamedly based on the Mediterranean Diet—because it is observed, by very good medical studies, to work. I have just updated it in light of new advances. I find it simple, pleasant, easy to remember and, yes, a gentle, diet—free of aggressive and didactic rules, processed foods, and strange additives from the factory.

There are, of course, some drugs that must be taken but even these can be minimized. Recently it has been found that the original heart risk calculators are now out of date and inaccurate; yet they have been used to put millions of people on drugs they didn't need.

And so it goes. It is up to you to accept responsibility and to act on it. You now have to become a Type 3 "Health Active Responsible" person (but I can live without you being "intense and demanding").

Patient Types and Outcomes

From the table below it can be seen that those who are most proactive achieve the best results:

Patient Type	**Response To Illness**	**Clinicians See Them**	**Health Outcome**
Type 1 **Passive**	Resigned	Unmotivated	Worst
Type 2 **Concerned**	Obedient	Cooperative But Overly Dependent	Average
Type 3 **Health Active Responsible**	Involved, Intense, Self-Directed	Motivated And Demanding	Best

For optimum health you have to be "health active and responsible." This means accepting responsibility for your own health and not expecting the government or someone else to look after you. It is your responsibility to exercise, eat healthy foods and to find out the known evidence for successful aging. It is your responsibility to study the Death and Disability tables, take specific avoidance actions and get tested.

All this is documented in ***Live Longest***... but the ball is in your court—you are effectively on your own. This does not mean help is not at hand; but it does mean no one else can exercise or eat for you or cut out your high-risk behaviors. I am not blind or immune to the fact that smoking is a most wretched addiction, incredibly difficult to give up; and so is overeating and eating the wrong foods; but the choice is yours. Go sit on a mountain and think it through. You can die prematurely or be disabled 20 years before you should, or you can adopt the world's best-evidenced medical advice.

If sitting on a mountain doesn't convince you, go visit a nursing home.

But hey! It ain't all that bad! In fact you will never feel better while living the best lifestyle possible. This is not a punitive, spartan, madly disciplined regime, but rather proven, moderate (gentle) good sense.

The essence is to now know what is bad and replacing it with what is good, knowing what illnesses are most likely for your age and how to avoid them.

27. Compression Of Morbidity: Healthier Longer vs Sicker Longer

Increase Health Span, not Life Span

In 1980, Dr. James F. Fries, a Stanford University physician who studied chronic disease and aging, proposed that a "compression of morbidity" would enable most people to remain healthy until a certain age, perhaps 85, then die naturally or after only a brief illness.

While diverse strategies—from caloric restriction to genetic manipulation—have proven to extend life span in model organisms in the lab, these animals are not necessarily enjoying longer periods of health. Increasing lifespan also increases the acceleration of the age-dependent mortality rate of the population.

The "Future Ideal" is *Compression of Morbidity*—living healthier longer (with a good quality of life) by preventing age-related disease and physical decline. While minor progress is being made to try and reverse aging, this goal will be years away. What can be done immediately, however, is the predicting and therefore the preventing or minimizing of these disorders and illnesses, which is the practical purpose and objective of this book.

Avoid the Nursing Home!

Although people are now living longer, they are not necessarily healthier than before. Many people are "dying longer"—being kept alive without much quality of life. "Health span does not match up with lifespan." Nearly a quarter (23%) of the overall global burden of death and illness is in people aged over 60, and much of this burden is attributable to long-term illness caused by diseases such as cancer, chronic respiratory diseases, heart disease, musculoskeletal diseases (such as arthritis and osteoporosis), mental and neurological disorders. This long-term burden of illness and diminished wellbeing affects patients, their families, health systems, and economies, and is forecast to accelerate. For example, the latest estimates indicate that the number of people with dementia is expected to rise from 44 million now, to 135 million by 2050.[83]

We all must age, and in doing so, incur some unavoidable changes such as our hair whitening, our eyesight reducing, and the loss of muscle (sarcopenia). Many of these changes can be disguised or minimized. Elderly women look quite smart with hair dyed to look natural and not with grey streaks; laser surgery can make spectacles a thing of the past; and regular exercise minimizes muscle loss. Even so, we are not the same healthy bouncing ball we were at 11 years old; inevitably, we will incur some impost. The aim today, and a key point to this book, is to minimize any such imposts and live longer, being healthy, fit, functional, alert and independent.

I am not sure of this acronym but it may work for you: "HAFFI" - Healthy, Alert, Fit, Functioning, Independent.

The key is "Reduction in Morbidity" at the end of our lifespan. This means reducing the years of illness or disability by increasing the years of good health—"living healthier longer." At present the last 20 years or so of our lives, from 63 to 80 years of age, can be spent with some disability, usually in a nursing home or as a housebound vegetable. People are increasingly being "placed" in nursing homes and hospices with no control over their own lives.

There is almost a universal lack of official government programs to address this problem with evidenced prevention. Karelia in Finland, where government intervention reduced the highest rate of heart attacks to the least in Europe, is one of the very few I can find. So, it can be done; but usually all that happens are oodles of conferences attended by delegates paid to wring their hands over the fact that society is getting fatter and obesity is an epidemic. Or, as in Ireland, initial encouraging improvements soon relapse into the bad old ways of junk food, cigarettes, and illegal drugs, with no need to accept personal responsibility.

It can only get worse with the prediction of a future nightmare that, while we clever doctors keep us alive longer, into our 90s or beyond, this duration of invalid morbidity will exceed 40 years... but with not enough taxpayers to fund our care.

The frightening scenario that we all see every day is society getting fatter. The diseases of affluence follow this inexorable, predictable sequence: Affluence—greater leisure—affordable junk food—obesity—arthritis / back pain—increasing sedentary behavior—diabetes 2—heart disease—atrial fibrillation—depression—Alzheimer's... all of which the drug companies and the health scammers are only too eager to exploit. The costs are absolutely incredible... as are the profits to Big Pharma (see chapter 17).

It has been said that "society progresses on the backs of middle class morality." Now it is sustained by the taxes of those paying for this epidemic of diabetic drug(s), blood glucose testers, arthritis pills, cardiovascular disease medications, statins, PPIs, hospitalization, heart tests, anticoagulants, pacemakers, antidepressants, and then the caregivers and the nursing home expenses. Meanwhile the hospital doors, examination / operating tables and airplane seats have to be widened and reinforced.

Many of the patients I see are on 10 different drugs when, arguably, if they were lean and ate correctly they may not need any!

If you think I am being severe, please note what American cardiologist John Mandrola said in "Heart Disease and Lifestyle: Why Are Doctors in Denial?" (2015):

> I know that exercise, diet, sleep, and finding balance in life are the key components of success. It is the same in cardiology... but... Bulging waistlines, thick necks, sagging muscles, and waddling gaits have begun to look like normal. I rarely click on "normal" (for the) physical exam. The general appearance is abnormal—either overweight or obese. New anticoagulant drugs are easy. Ablation technology is easy. Statins are even easier. The truth—nutrition, exercise, and balance in life—is hard.[84]

Compression of Morbidity:
Now, Future Ideal, Future Nightmare

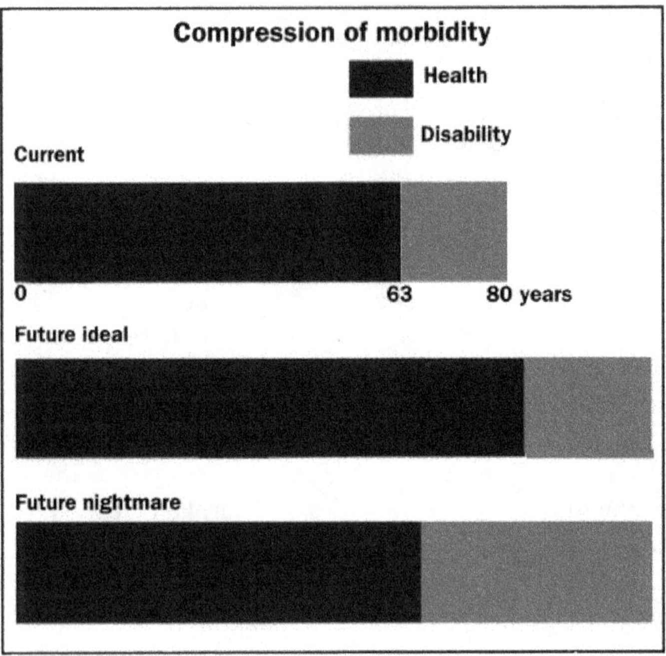

This "future, or indeed present, nightmare" need not be the case. But help is pretty thin on the ground. The politicians are too scared to implement preventive programs, such as reducing the taxes of those who are not obese, who are normotensive and with a normal biochemical profile. The doctors are only reimbursed for prescribing drugs or doing procedures. Patients expect prescriptions rather than advice. The drug companies have vested interests in not curing anyone. The vitamin/supplement factories make unsubstantiated claims which we believe. And finally, the commercial fast-food industry has an income that exceeds the GNP of most countries and is dedicated to getting you to eat their researched-to-be-delicious junk. A recent study done at Kiel University, Germany found both healthy and unhealthy consumers make their eating decisions based on taste alone. Despite being given information about the ingredients, this was not sufficient to encourage choosing the healthier food.[85]

I am not being critical, let alone superior, here. These are observed facts. It is human nature. But if we want to avoid being sicker longer we have to know these facts, be given the correct information and then an acceptable plan to avoid detrimental lifestyles, foods and habits.

To compress morbidity we must optimize our health. In doing so we optimize aging successfully and live longer.

NOTE: Our normal lifespan is pretty well fixed at present and cannot yet be prolonged or extended by much. When I say "live longer" I mean "don't die prematurely, but live your whole entitled lifespan"—something too many are not achieving because of the lack of essential medical information and advice, as documented in this book.

I hasten to say I do not claim to have discovered any secret fads ensuring longevity, nor to be the only person aware of these problems and solutions. Obviously there are many medical practitioners who are as aware as I am, and who know as much if not more; but they are either too busy as clinicians or too specialized.

The problem is shafted home in all its acute reality when patients are fat, unfit, have to be helped onto the examination couch, moaning and groaning, on a dozen or so different medications. In addition there are of course, the epidemiologists, social economists who see and predict the overall economic and social problems; and then there are the researchers and PhDs who provide the valuable statistics. But we all lack the resources and mechanisms to fix it... to compress this morbidity.

It is and will be your personal responsibility to adopt the healthiest lifestyle.

This book provides the best information available to date on how to do so.

Doctors Only Attend the Ill

Historically, medical practitioners were only sought if and when people were ill. Thus health schemes, whether introduced by government or insurance companies, were based on remunerating the doctor for treating these recognized illnesses. Doctors were not reimbursed for preventing illnesses and thus moved into areas of medicine where they could see results and would get paid. Not only has prevention languished but also doctors have become de-skilled in this area.

Because clinicians can only treat individuals after illnesses are established, they simply do not practice prevention or evidenced good health advice. This has created a vacuum and allowed the zealots, charlatans, beauty therapists, gym, health food and vitamin industries to sweep in and "round up the usual suspects"—the people, like you, desperate to be healthy while largely being given the wrong advice.

Personal Responsibility

The greatest obstruction to good medical prevention and health care is you... especially if you are a male. Men don't go to doctors... and guess what? Men die 4 or more years before women. It used to be 7 years. Men aren't improving; women are smoking more and indulging in higher risk behaviors.

Most people would prefer to spend their money on a new car, plasma TV, holidays, restaurants, wine, their home or clothes... which is certainly more pleasant than having a fiber-optic cable threaded up your colon, a finger up your rectum or your breasts compressed between two steel plates. And I am one of them!

But we can't enjoy a new car, LED TV, holidays, restaurants, wine, home, clothes or even your family *unless we are well!*

No one knows how to inspire you to get these done (a heart attack is one of the best ways... if you survive). But if you commit to preventive maintenance it will follow proven guidelines for lifestyle changes and diagnostic tests. There is no rebate for servicing or repairing your car or for cosmetic surgery. If you do have to pay for some of these tests for which there is little rebate and the test results come back clear, then it would seem that this is money not just well spent, but best spent!

Surveys rate Health at No. 1 for Successful Aging

Where the Health Budgets Go

Modeling in 2015 by Avid Culen, chief economist at the Australian Commonwealth Department of Health, showed that changes in age structure between 1915 and 2010 have only made a small contribution to the recent growth in health expenditure, with less than 10% of the net increment in per capita health spending explained by demography.[86]

However, if the health systems stay the same, the aging population will increase the health expenditure on this age group to a third of the total. Even now a 75-year-old costs some $500 more each year than a 70-year-old.

The problem is multifactorial, with each "factor" pursuing their own ends and, to a degree, vested interests. In my observation this has led to an explosion in hospitals as the main cause of health cost blowouts. Politicians love them, as they are often claiming them as monuments to their tenure and dubious achievements. Specialists love them, as it gives legitimacy to procedures such as expensive joint replacements in the very old: the surgeon earns money, the hospital earns money, the surgical supply company earns money, the hospital nurses, wardsmen, clerks, engineers, gardeners, and laundry staff all get paid from these operations and procedures. Then there are the end-of-life chemotherapies, which are not necessary, or even contra-indicated, and the politician, where the governments subsidize health care and hospitals, bathes in the reflected glory, claiming to have delivered health to his or her constituency.

As pointed out in the 2015 report on the inquiry into skin cancer in Australia, "early treatment following early diagnosis can reduce the cost of treatment from $3000 in a public hospital to $300 in a skin cancer clinic,"[87] and $11,323 in a USA hospital compared with $1,745 as an out patient In other words, a private skin clinic is 10 times more cost-efficient.

My estimate, just to be admitted overnight and sit on a hospital bed without anything being done is between $1000 and $4000.

While there are obviously certain procedures that can only be done in hospitals, the exploitation or misuse of GPs and primary care doctors worldwide (as above), combined with the increase in medical litigation, has resulted in them simply sloughing many problems, no matter how minor, to the hospitals, whose legal bills are simply incredible. I know because the lawyer for one very big teaching hospital is a patient of mine, and a recent news article says the same about NHS hospitals in the UK.

The blowout in medical litigation has forced defensive medical practices such as ordering a CT scan for a headache just to placate a patient. It has become so ridiculous that any disturbed person can make a frivolous and mischievous complaint about a doctor who then has to spend inordinate stressful time defending him or herself while the complainant is not penalized if found to be frivolous.

One excellent doctor I know had a complaint because a patient demanded he do an operation then and there. While this complaint was eventually thrown out, the stress was such that my colleague had a heart attack and retired from medicine.

The worldwide denigration and exploitation of primary care has simply resulted in passive resistance by GPs and the resultant unchecked expansion of unchecked hospital costs. No politician will prevent a 90-year-old having a hip replacement, as they want the votes.

CT scan, anyone? Unnecessary operations when you want, anyone?

Meanwhile back at primary care, where most people go to get health advice: "There is no other part of the health care system that is in greater trouble right now... The typical work day of a primary Care Physician (a GP in Australia and the United Kingdom) in the early 21st century is built on seeing as many patients as possible in the office in a given day... Insurers (and Governments) financially motivate PCPs to keep patient visits brief."[88]

This is also why preventive medicine is not practiced, let alone pursued and updated, as are all other advances in medicine.

Not Whining

All is not well in the hospitals either: Two of our most vital industries, health care and education, have become increasingly subjected to metrics and measurements. Of course, we need to hold professionals accountable. But the focus on numbers has gone too far. We're hitting the targets, but missing the point...

A 2013 study found that the electronic health record was a dominant culprit. Another 2013 study found that emergency room doctors clicked a mouse 4,000 times during a 10-hour shift. The computer systems have become the dark force behind quality measures... In medicine, doctors no longer made eye contact with patients as they clicked away. Thoughtful and limited assessment can be effective in motivating improvements and innovations (but) we need to tone down the fervor and think harder about the unanticipated consequences. We need to appreciate the burden that measurement places on professionals to minimize it.[89]

Competition for the Health Dollar: The Health Industry

"Health" has now become big business and is referred to as a "product." Patients are now "consumers." It is predicted to be the next trillion-dollar industry, if it's not already. As such, there is enormous competition for the health dollar, *your dollar,* from the following health-interested parties:

Who wants your health dollar?

In order...

1. Governments
2. Insurers
3. Hospitals
4. Drug Companies
5. Food Industry
6. Tobacco Industry
7. Media
8. Doctors
9. Allied health professionals
10. Health workers
11. Patients (now "consumers")
12. Complementary and Alternative Medicine (CAM)
13. Health farms and spas
14. Business
15. Supply and service companies

Of these, somewhat remarkably and surprisingly, it is the fast-food industry, with a US turnover in the trillions of dollars—bigger than the GDP of most countries—which has arguably the most direct influence on our health.

The blame for the obesity epidemic and its sequela of the metabolic syndrome cannot be laid entirely at the feet of the fast-food industry; but given that our food has changed more in the last 40 years than in the previous 40,000,[90] it must certainly be considered a prime suspect.

We now live in a toxic food environment where some 4,000 to 6,000 calories a day are produced for every man, woman and child, when we need less than 2,000.

It is a somewhat frightening realization that the patient and the doctor have practically the least say in how we are being manipulated by most of the above.

How Then to Get the Correct Care to the People Who Want It?

The above is only to alert you to the running interference, health budgets, competition for your health dollar and problems which make accessing the best medical treatment, advice and information progressively difficult. At the very top level, the system works brilliantly. We have never had it so good at this level. MRIs, organ transplants, artificial limbs, artificial aortas, cochlear implants, heart valves replaced and normal rhythm restored "while you wait." Meanwhile, preventive medicine has languished and never realized its potential; and given this interference, it most likely never will. So "what can a poor fella do?"

Here is the ***Live Longest*** contribution. It is ruthlessly honest, without the hype of fads. It provides the latest independent evidence, proven by the best-referenced trials. These trials have a huge sample of people (some over 100,000) and cover many years; and the results are blinded and interpreted by independent persons.

Insurance Cover

The type and level of a person's health insurance affects access to screening. One American study reported that only 32.7% of uninsured people were screened for colorectal cancer, versus. 53.2% of those insured. A survey reported middle-aged English people were healthier than their American cohorts and inferred that access to Britain's free NHS was the reason. There may be a case for only doing colonoscopies on symptomatic patients, but colonoscopy is a routine test for presidents of the United States and saved Ronald Reagan's life.

Implementation Difficulties

Proof does not always ensure implementation, as we know from such ostensibly simple, achievable, effective and evidenced pieces of preventive medicine as reducing salt below 7 g a day in people with hypertension, and minimizing sugar intake. The reduction in salt would have a large effect on reducing strokes and heart attacks in predisposed people, as excess salt represents the greatest preventable cause of worsening hypertension. Seventy-five percent of salt comes from processed food. Most of this is in bread and breakfast cereals; but reducing it in processed food is unachievable on a large scale because of government reluctance to interfere with big business. After all, wars have been fought and empires lost over salt.[91] Not all salt is bad (see the Newtrition Notes); the problem is that it's being added to food and people are not really aware how much of it they are eating.

Costs

When doctors in the United Kingdom were no longer paid to perform circumcisions, the procedure suddenly became a "mutilation" and any doctors who tried to point out the possible benefits were howled down. I know because I had done research into STDs, and when specializing in Edinburgh, the professor of pediatric surgery was incredibly rude and arrogant (and wrong) when I mildly suggested that circumcision may have some benefits. Some 50 years on, it has been found that circumcision significantly protects against HIV-AIDS, HBV (cervical cancer), other infections and even cancer of the prostate, and will soon be "recommended" as it now is in South Africa and is (and was) cost effective.

As documented most Preventive Measures are, or can be, cheap.

Complementary and Alternative Medicine (CAM)

All these impediments to good medicine have opened the door for the entrepreneurs, charlatans, mountebanks and misguided zealots who seized the preventive health high ground with vitamins, minerals, health foods and weight clinics, as well as the fringe anti-aging medicine of growth hormones and unproven therapeutics. Western medical graduates were perceived as not providing "holistic" (a Western medicine word) care; whereas CAM promoted so-called "natural" cures. Sixty percent of people now admit to using alternate therapies. But much is a waste of money. Large, international very well conducted trials have found that not only do multivitamin and antioxidant supplements not work, but they can also shorten our lives. Vitamins are necessary if we are malnourished; otherwise they are best obtained from natural foods. It is always tragically amusing to me to see advocates of "natural CAM" taking unnatural vitamins and supplements made in a factory. There are some 83,000 health supplements on sale in the United States. Only 13 vitamins are necessary for our health and all of these are available from food (fruit, vegetables, meat and sunshine) in the correct dose. The National Health Statistics Report reveals that Americans now spend up to $34 billion dollars per year on complementary alternative medicine.

I have an open mind, or try to. After all, aspirin came from the bark of the willow tree, and digitalis from the foxglove; while penicillin was a mould on bread and fruit. These may well be considered "natural" and "alternative," but the difference is that they have been subjected to extraction of the pure active substance and then endless animal experiments and trials before the correct dose and side effects are known and released to the public. In **Book 2 Newtrition** I expand on the **Micronutrient Revolution** - the 6000(+), mostly phytonutrients, which have evidenced profound health benefits - available in our every day, easily obtainable foods - if you know which is which.

I even learned acupuncture from the London doctor, Felix Mann, who brought it out of China and first introduced it to the West. It works on selected cases and for some quite remarkably well. However, CAM is mostly a waste of money, allowing the quacks and charlatans to sell snake oil or its equivalents. Unlike Western medicine, there are no evidenced trials and, of course, the placebo effect is about 60% positive.

I recently listened to a remarkable talk on my car radio. It was a woman writer who had a wonderful, enviable style that captured me and prevented me changing stations. It evolved she was poor, suffering some illness and, despite her apparent dogged resilience, she bemoaned the fact that she had spent so much, "a small fortune," on useless alternative therapies such as paw-paw wraps, which was why she was now so poor. The announcer came on after the program to identify her and say she died from multiple sclerosis in 2009.

Excuse me if I am suffused with disgust and loathing for these scam artists who so defraud such vulnerable people while seducing them with false hopes. Paw-paw oil is just a meat tenderizer enzyme, papain. It had a big vogue in the 60s for treating "slipped discs." The FDA banned it so

Americans flocked like lemmings up to Canada where the doctors made a fortune injecting their spinal discs. The FDA was correct—it doesn't work.

My only CAM at present is an interest in curcumin and inulin. Tumeric / curcumin has long been associated with a possible reduction in cancer. Inulin, usually from the root of chicory, is associated with reduced visceral fat. Some doctors also recommend magnesium, about which we know very little.

Socioeconomic Dichotomy

Socioeconomic status is a combination of education, income and occupation. A person may be a slum orphan but a business or scientific genius and so is considered as Class I, whereas some hereditary aristocrat may be a bumbling fool and drops down the scale. One working system for health delivery is:

Class I: Professional and higher managerial

Class II: Intermediate

Class III: Small employers and own account workers

Class IV: Supervisors, craft-related, and skilled manual workers

Class V: Working class, unskilled

The Failure of Free Health

The health interest in these groups is that the poorer groups are ostensibly denied access to good, let alone the best, health care. In the United Kingdom, the introduction of a national health scheme, in the late 1940s, allowed the poor free access to all the the twentieth-century advances, improvements and benefits to health—the identification of the importance of germs, the introduction of hygiene, anesthesia and sterile surgery, x-rays, antibiotics, more and more hospitals, better drugs, tests and better trained doctors. They could now access *free consultations, free medicine and free operations.*

Surely now it would be reasonable to conclude that these poorer classes would at last enjoy better health and that their health should now equal that of the richer classes.

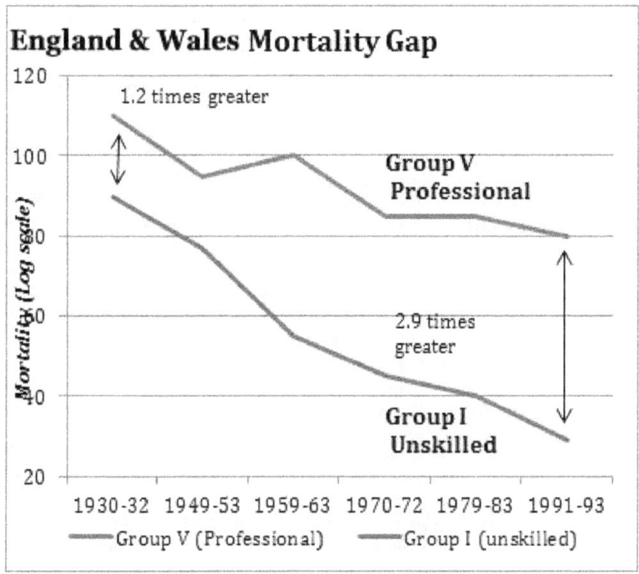

Between 1930 and 1990, despite the best medical treatments, tests, investigations, and medicines, hospitals and operations being offered and supplied ***for free,*** from the late 1940s, the unskilled classes' health in the United Kingdom has become nearly three times worse than that of the more affluent class.

Free health doesn't work. You have to get the right information and then do it yourself.

Since 1930 the mortality of the poorer classes has become worse, from 1.2 to 2.9 times worse than socioeconomic Class I, despite free medicine, hospitals and all advances.

A University of Oxford study reported in 2006: "The poorest children in the United Kingdom, those born into the lowest socioeconomic group, have a 40% increased chance of dying in the first 10 years of life compared with children born into the highest socioeconomic group."

It would seem that the poorer and less-educated socioeconomic classes are both ill-informed and not motivated to take responsibility for their health.

The Strategic Policy Unit Report for the Australian Health Minister (August 2014) found that morbidity, or disease, occurs more often in poor households (2.6 times the rate in the richest); in communities with the least education (1.2 times the rate in the most educated); in unemployed groups (3.1 times the rate for those who have jobs); and in remote areas (1.4 times the rate of those living in major cities). Premature death is also more common among those disadvantaged groups. Every percentage point difference in the number of adults facing financial stress corresponds to an increase of about 4 premature deaths for every 100,000 people.[92]

This data, of course, is not meant to impute or demean any attempts to deliver people health care. It does, however, call into question the present efficiency of national health schemes no matter how well intentioned. Government agencies, even the WHO, spend millions upon millions annually on producing pretty posters, booklets, handouts and even running TV advice, but with little results. The waste of money is an obscenity and could arguably be better spent.

While responsibility for health is up to the individual, given the enormous resources set against us—feeding us misinformation; bent on extracting our health dollar; advertising fast foods, vitamins, alcohol and in some countries, even smoking—we don't stand a chance unless we consult the world's best, uncorrupted, independent studies.

I hasten to add that I do not regard these different groups fighting for the health dollar as sinister. They have merely filled a vacuum left by legitimate evidenced medicine. A gullible, uninformed public has embraced the false claims and advertising and even prefers it to the correct advice. As will be seen in **Book 2: "Newtrition"**, healthy foods are never labeled "healthy." If a supermarket has a "Healthy" or "Health" food section, what does that make the rest of the foods? The advertising industry assures us this or that breakfast mix is "healthy," and the fast-food industry makes it delicious and therefore preferable to unprocessed, natural foods... meanwhile it's just a pity about the high sodium, sugar and fat content that makes it so delicious (but deadly). And so, the fast-food chains, the vitamin and supplement manufacturers, and so on are pandering to (and exploiting) a demand. They are not the moral or health guardians of society.

Finally, it should be noted that despite seemingly heavy burdens of disease and illness, many people, such as Franklin Roosevelt and Stephen Hawking, have managed to carry major health infirmities and still achieve success and contribute mightily to society.

Can Compression of Morbidity Be Achieved?

While most people struggle with an ever-increasing burden of disease and disability as they age, it has been found that those who live exceptionally long lives have the additional benefit of shorter periods of illness—sometimes just weeks or months—before death. These findings suggest that discoveries made in one group of centenarians can be generalized to diverse populations. And they contradict the notion that the older people get, the sicker they become and the greater the cost of taking care of them.[93]

Four General Barometers That Help Define Healthy Behavior (but Only 2.7% of Americans Do So):

1. Good diet
2. Moderate exercise
3. Recommended body fat percentage
4. Non-smoker

Such characteristics are associated with a lower risk of most serious illnesses but only 2.7% of the US adult population achieves all four of these basic behavioral characteristics that would constitute a "healthy lifestyle."[94]

28. Universal Advice

A Note On Cholesterol

Cardiovascular Disease (heart attacks and strokes) are the greatest cause of premature death and disabilities in all Western societies, and has been subject to some recent controversy, so this is addressed at the outset.

In the 1960s Finnish men had the world's highest death rate from heart disease. They liked butter and lard on their bread, and also favored whole milk, cheese, salt, sausage, and cigarettes. Only occasionally did they eat fruit or vegetables, saying this was "food for animals." In 1972 the Karelia Project introduced what was essentially a Mediterranean Diet, and by the early 2000s, for men aged from 35 to 64, the number of deaths from coronary heart disease had plunged about 75%—probably the most dramatic and best population-wide improvement yet recorded. Much of this reduction is attributed to dramatic reductions in risk factors like high blood pressure, high cholesterol and smoking. Lowered cholesterol was attributed as the strongest contributor.

This information is enlarged and discussed in detail in the **Newtrition** book.

Recently there are emerging studies that show how eating saturated fat and having high cholesterol is okay and even beneficial.[47] I have an open mind and will watch for future studies. But while these latest articles may "welcome" fat and having high cholesterol, for a doctor like me who was running a coronary care unit and seeing middle-aged men dying prematurely from heart attacks in the late 60s early 70s, I still regard the Karelia Project with undiminished admiration. So I stick to the ***Newtrition PHYTO Diet (Book 2)***—the Mediterranean-based diet like the one the Finns adopted to lower their heart attack rates from the worst to the best rates in the world.

It strikes me the medical profession will now divide into two camps, those advocating low cholesterol even if it means taking statins, and the new group saying saturated fat and high cholesterol is okay or even good. Both, however, still encourage lifestyle changes (no smoking, more exercise, BP control).

In the following two chapters it is recommended that you get your lipid (especially LDL cholesterol) levels done. I would still do this but, due to this recent challenge, you should be guided by your own doctor.

As I have pointed out, medicine has vogues but eventually the truth is revealed. In the meantime I will stick to and recommend my ***Newtrition PHYTO Diet (Book 2)***, as this approach has had some 60 years of documented benefit. But I don't get uptight if I eat the occasional saturated fat. It is now apparent that not all saturated fats behave the same in the body. Some fat sources are actually beneficial, and unsaturated oils are still better overall than saturated fats.

Butter would seem to be "neutral." A study found only weak or neutral effects of butter consumption on overall mortality and cardiovascular disease (CVD) risk, suggesting that butter may not be as harmful as previously thought, and may not be as harmful as the white bread and potatoes it is spread on.[48]

However, eating higher amounts of saturated and trans fat increases the risk for death, while eating polyunsaturated fats (PUFAs) and monounsaturated fats (MUFAs) may lower the risk of death. Replacing saturated fats with the same amount of calories from Polys and Monos was linked to a reduced risk for overall death. A total of 84,349 women from the Nurses' Health Study and 42,884 men from the Health Professionals Follow-up Study, over 32 years of follow-up results, showed increased risk of death with consumption of saturated and trans fats. Polys and Monos were linked to a reduced risk of death.[49]

This study of 127,233 health professionals followed for 32 years is, to me, just as significant, if not more so, as the North Karaelia Project and what I recommend in Newtrition PHYTO Diet (Book 2).

Stroke Risk Factors

Ten modifiable risk factors responsible for 90% of strokes[50]

Stroke is a highly preventable disease globally, regardless of age and sex. Ten modifiable risk factors are associated with 90% of stroke cases in all world regions, younger and older and in men and women. The two major types of stroke include ischaemic stroke caused by blood clots, which accounts for 85% of strokes, and haemorrhagic stroke or bleeding into the brain, which accounts for 15% of strokes.

Hypertension is the most important modifiable risk factor. The number of strokes would be practically cut in half (48%) if hypertension was eliminated; trimmed by more than a third (36%) if people were physically active; and shaved by almost one fifth (19%) if they had better diets. In addition, this proportion was cut back by 12% if smoking was eliminated; 9% for cardiac (heart) causes, 4% for diabetes, 6% for alcohol intake, 6% for stress, and 27% for lipids (the study used apolipoproteins, which was found to be a better predictor of stroke than total cholesterol). When combined together, the total for all 10 risk factors was 91%, which was similar in all regions, age groups and in men and women.

% Stroke Reduction

48% if hypertension controlled

36% if people were physically active

27% for lipid control

19% with better diets

12% if smoking was eliminated

9% for cardiac causes (Atrial Fibrillation)

6% for alcohol intake

6% for stress

4% for diabetes

Atrial fibrillation, an irregular heart rhythm, was significantly associated with ischaemic stroke in all regions, but was of greater importance in Western Europe, North America and Australia, than in China or South Asia.

Air Pollution and Strokes

Each year around the world, approximately 15 million people have a stroke. Of these, 6 million die and 5 million are left permanently disabled, making stroke the second leading cause of disability.

A recent study implicates air pollution as a leading risk factor for stroke worldwide with about 30% of the global stroke burden is due to air pollution. Pollution includes environmental and household air pollution. Some 30% of disability associated with stroke is linked to air pollution, which is especially high in developing countries compared with developed countries, at 33.7% and 10.2%, respectively.

The study also provided information on the contribution of all 17 risk factors for stroke. The top five risk factors for stroke in the UK and USA were:

1. high blood pressure
2. high BMI
3. diet low in fruit
4. diet low in vegetables
5. smoking.[51]

Burning coal has the worst health impact of any source of air pollution and is responsible for the deadly fine particulate matter known as PM 2.5, contributing to 2.9 million premature deaths worldwide, with 64% of those in China, India and other developing countries in Asia and also in Eastern Europe.[52]

Now toxic magnetite nanoparticles from air pollution have been discovered in human brains in abundant quantities. They are formed as molten droplets of material from combustion sources, such as car exhaust, industrial processes and power stations, anywhere there is burning fuel. Magnetite is everywhere: an analysis of roadside air in Lancaster found 200 million magnetite particles per cubic meter. There is no blood-brain barrier when inhaled through the nose. It is conjectured that this may be a cause of Alzheimer's disease, as an impaired sense of smell is an early indicator of Alzheimer's disease.[53]

Smoking

Smoking is incredibly injurious to our health and arguably the most pervasive of all drugs of addiction. It is essential to quit.

Cigarettes liberate 6,000 substances of which 100 are known to be injurious to us. It has been found that to quit, people need support. Nicotine replacement at present offers the best results, while e-cigarettes are promising as they seem to cause 95% less damage, though their long-term effects are not known.

Suicide and Older White Men

Older white men have higher suicide rates, yet fewer burdens associated with aging. For example, they are less likely to experience death of a spouse and have better physical health and fewer disabilities than older women. They have more economic resources than ethnic minority older men and women. White older men, however, may be less psychologically equipped to deal with the normal challenges of aging because of their privilege up until late adulthood. It is thought that an important factor in white men's psychological brittleness and vulnerability to suicide once they reach late life may be the belief that suicide is a masculine response to the "indignities" of aging. This is a script that implicitly justifies, and even glorifies, suicide among men as a rational, courageous, powerful choice. Two such famous cases were Eastman Kodak founder George Eastman, who died of suicide in 1932 at age 77—it was said he was "unprepared and unwilling to face the indignities of old age"—and Gonzo-writer Hunter S. Thompson, who killed himself in 2005 at age 67, having thus triumphed over "the indignities of aging." But older men are not the most suicide-prone group everywhere. For example, in China, women of reproductive age are the group with the highest suicide mortality. The "indignities of aging" suicide script as well as the belief that suicide is a white man's powerful response to aging can and should be challenged, and changed.

Suicides in the United States increased 24% from 1999 to 2014, according to data from the CDC. This rate increased from 1% to 2% annually from 2006 through 2014, a timespan that included the Great Recession. The female suicide rate increased 45% since 1999 and the male suicide rate increased 16%. Nonetheless, in 2014, the age-adjusted suicide rate among males was still 3 times that in females (20.7 vs. 5.8 per 100,000). Suicide rates were highest in men aged 75 and older and in women aged 45–64. In children aged 10–14, suicide rates were low, but this age group had a large percentage increase in suicides (200% in females, 37% in males). About a quarter of suicides are attributed to suffocation, an increase since 1999. For men, the most frequent method involved firearms. For women, poisoning was the most common method.[54]

ON YER BIKE

Cycling to work has been shown to have profound benefits better than walking: People who reported biking to work had a lower risk for all-cause mortality, compared with people who drove or took public transportation. Cycling was also tied to reduced risks for both CVD incidence and mortality and cancer incidence and mortality. Walking was associated only with reduced cardiovascular risk.[7]

[7] Association between active commuting and incident cardiovascular disease, cancer, and mortality: prospective cohort study BMJ 2017;357:j1456

29. Studies and Trials

How They Are Done and Their Relative Significance and Value

Studies and trials are done in different ways, with increasingly better methods, results and evidence. Their terminology is bandied about such that they may seem more important than they actually are, so it's handy for you to know the basics. The gold standard is the Double Blind Randomized Controlled Trial (RCT).

The pecking order is:

Observation: This is where an association of circumstances may be linked to an illness or a benefit. Obviously, there are both high- and low-standard studies.

The classic example is the ancient Romans, who thought fog caused malaria. Indeed, when Caesar drained the Pontine Marshes and there was no fog, there was no malaria. This was *observation and association*; later studies found it was a blood parasite and later studies found it was carried by mosquitoes.

Any benefits or harm from foods or diets are mostly observational studies.

Observational studies can only document associations; they cannot demonstrate causation. Moreover, the measurement error in epidemiologic studies of diet and disease is often significant. These measurement errors often bias the associations toward the null (invalid-useless), making it possible that health effects are being missed.

Case report: is where a description of a patient's or a series of patients' illness can generate a hypothesis; but this cannot be tested, as there is no comparison group.

Clinical trial: An experimental study where the exposure of patients or participants to a drug or a causative agent is determined by the investigator(s).

Cohort study: A cohort is simply a group of often similar people. These are observational studies but done over time to subjects or participants exposed to the object of the study (e.g., fiber in the diet). Results are then compared with subjects not so exposed (no fiber).

Cross-sectional study: An observational study where participants are assessed as to the effect of an exposure. This is somewhat historical, as the exposure and outcome are determined at the same time; so it is unclear if the exposure preceded the outcome.

Randomized controlled trial (RCT): Participants are assigned purely by chance to an exposure.

Double Blind RCT: The gold standard. The participants are chosen randomly without anyone knowing their identity—the selectors are "blinded." The exposing agent (e.g., a drug) is doubled with an identical looking placebo, and again the administrator does not know which is which. Finally, the results are assessed by analysists who have also been blinded (i.e., the whole way, no one knows which is which, who is who or what is what, and the results are therefore completely innocent, uninfluenced and independent.

The best trials make it into the best medical journals (for which there is also a pecking order) after they have been peer reviewed (i.e., reviewed by experts in that subject as to their worth). Only the best trials and journals have been consulted and used for this book.

Statistics are a problem the magnitude of which is, I feel, just being realized. Trial after trial has utilized and manipulated statistics to support what the study authors want and not what is correct. All studies now have to show statistics. The most used value is ***P*, signifying probability**, or the value for the threshold of significance. For example, a probability value $P < 0.05$ assures us that the result is significant. The next is **Confidence Intervals**, which, by convention, are set at 95%, which suggests the true population value is represented. **Confounders** are mixed effects, where there are other factors which may mask and alter the results. For example, it may be found that eating a certain food was associated with increased running speed; but what if these subjects were fit, young, non-smoking, healthy athletes? Would the same food have worked on the fat, old, smoking and unfit?

30. Big Pharma

Most of us, including doctors, have no idea of the incredible expenditure (and profits) involved with drugs. Most drugs, of course, are necessary, and many desirable; but the pharmaceutical companies (Big Pharma) who often pay for these trails have frequently hidden any bad results. One of the worst examples was MSD and their drug Vioxx, which caused heart attacks; the manufacturer suppressed this information and 84,000 Vioxx-taking patients died from heart attacks until it was withdrawn.

All drugs have side effects, so if you can minimize them, do so.

100 Best-Selling, Most Prescribed Branded Drugs in the United States Through June 2015

Through June of 2015, the cholesterol-lowering drug rosuvastatin (*Crestor*, AstraZeneca) was the most prescribed branded drug in the United States, and the arthritis drug adalimumab (*Humira*, Abbott Laboratories) was the best-selling branded drug, according to the latest data from research firm IMS Health.

Rosuvastatin had about 21 million prescriptions, followed by asthma medication fluticasone propionate/salmeterol (*Advair Diskus*, GlaxoSmithKline), at about 13.6 million prescriptions; the proton pump inhibitor esomeprazole (*Nexium*, AstraZeneca), at about 13.2 million prescriptions; the insulin glargine injection *Lantus Solostar* (sanofi-aventis), at about 11.2 million; and the attention deficit drug lisdexamfetamine dimesylate (*Vyvanse*, Shire), at about 10.6 million.

Rounding out the top 10 most prescribed drugs for the period (in order) were the antiepileptic drug pregabalin (*Lyrica*, Pfizer), the chronic obstructive pulmonary disease medication tiotropium bromide (*Spiriva Handihaler*, Boehringer Ingelheim Pharmaceuticals), the diabetes drug sitagliptin (*Januvia*, Merck), the asthma/chronic obstructive pulmonary disease drug budesonide/formoterol (*Symbicort*, AstraZeneca), and the antipsychotic medication aripiprazole (*Abilify*, Otsuka Pharmaceutical).

Top Sellers

The top seller, arthritis drug adalimumab (*Humira*, Abbott Laboratories), had sales of about $8.6 billion, followed by the antipsychotic aripiprazole (*Abilify*, Otsuka Pharmaceutical), at $7.2 billion; the arthritis drug etanercept (*Enbrel*, Amgen), at roughly $6.1 billion; the cholesterol drug rosuvastatin (*Crestor*, AstraZeneca), at just under $6.1 billion; and the insulin glargine injection *Lantus Solostar* (sanofi-aventis), at around $5 billion.

The remaining top 10 drugs in sales were the hepatitis C drug sofosbuvir (*Sovaldi*, Gilead Sciences), at $4.9 billion; the asthma drug fluticasone propionate/salmeterol (*Advair Diskus*, GlaxoSmithKline), at $4.8 billion; the proton pump inhibitor esomeprazole (*Nexium*, AstraZeneca), at $4.7 billion; the diabetes drug sitagliptin (*Januvia*, Merck), at $3.8 billion; and the antiepileptic pregabalin (*Lyrica*, Pfizer), at $3.4 billion.

It is important to realize, given Big Pharma's track record of hiding bad results and persisting with killer drugs, that the moral and business principles that drive these drug companies are not always directed to peoples' health. A healthy suspicion of any new drug is advised. In essence they are developing products to make money. To get them to market is incredibly complex and expensive, with a number of audited phases to pass through. Only the very richest companies can afford this research and development. They are not there for the good of mankind. The object is making a profit; but to do so the product, the drug, should provide a benefit. Sometimes, however, deleterious side effects have been deliberately suppressed and hidden by the drug companies.

Businessmen who have a different moral compass than medical practitioners run these companies. Doctors (presumably) go into medicine to help people, whereas businessmen go into business to make money. I am not being holier-than-thou here, but pointing out essential differences which, if they concord, benefit all concerned; but when they don't, the drug companies have been known to put profit first and patient welfare last. Cholesterol-lowering statin drugs have been assessed as the most lucrative class of drugs ever sold in the history of mankind.

Top 100 Brands by Sales

Product (Trade name first, then Generic) – Sales, $

Humira: Adalimumab – for rheumatoid and other arthritis – **$8,566,451,647**

Abilify: Aripiprazole – an atypical antipsychotic for schizophrenia and bipolar disorder - $7,238,451,779

Enbrel: Etanercept – for autoimmune diseases – $6,139,812,530

Crestor: Rosuvastatin – a statin used to treat high cholesterol – $6,090,223,570

Lantus Solostar: Insulinglargine – injection for diabetes – $5,023,092,599

Sovaldi: Sofosbuvir – for the treatment of hepatitis C virus infection – $4,925,098,469

Advair Diskus: Fluticasone – for asthma – $4,769,250,836

Nexium: Esomeprazole – a proton pump inhibitor (PPI) used in the treatment of dyspepsia, peptic ulcer disease, gastroesophageal reflux disease – $4,709,542,900

Januvia: Sitagliptin – for diabetes 2 – $3,792,531,657

Lyrica: Pregabalin – used to treat epilepsy, neuropathic pain, fibromyalgia, and generalized anxiety disorder – $3,442,755,962

Spiriva Handihaler: Tiotropium – inhalation powder for asthma – $3,388,442,306

Symbicort: Budesonide and Formoterol – used to prevent bronchospasm in people with asthma or COPD – $2,480,108,204

Xarelto: Rivaroxaban – a novel (new) anticoagulant – $2,460,606,162

Vyvanse: Lisdexamfetamine – a central nervous system (CNS) stimulant used for ADHD and binge eating – $2,255,494,506

Novolog Flexpen: Insulin pen – delivery for diabetes – $2,212,204,664

Zetia: Ezetimibe – lowers plasma cholesterol levels by decreasing absorption – $2,155,848,498

Stelara: Ustekinumab – a monoclonal antibody used for immune system disorders and psoriasis – $1,781,288,922

Prevnar Pneumococcal vaccine – used to prevent infection caused by pneumococcal bacteria – $1,746,605,006

Humalog Kwikpen: Insulin – short duration for diabetes – $1,588,639,456

Gilenya: Fingolimod – an immunomodulating drug, mostly used for treating multiple sclerosis – $1,577,027,870

Cialis: Tadalafil – a PDE5 inhibitor marketed in pill form for treating erectile dysfunction – $1,520,551,442

Restasis: Cyclosporine – an immunosuppressant to prevent rejection n organ transplantation – $1,410,652,178

Latuda: Lurasidone – an atypical antipsychotic – $1,379,675,847

Viagra: Sildenafil – for erectile dysfunction and pulmonary arterial hypertension – $1,375,305,952

Seroquel XR: Quetiapine – an atypical antipsychotic for the treatment of schizophrenia, bipolar disorder, and along with an antidepressant to treat major depressive disorder – $1,359,121,073

Celebrex: Celecoxib – a Cox 2 nonsteroidal anti-inflammatory (NSAID) inhibitor for pain and inflammation for arthritis, acute pain, and menstrual pain and discomfort – $1,323,059,229

Invokana: Canagliflozin – a gliflozin class or subtype 2 sodium-glucose transport inhibitors used for the treatment of type 2 diabetes – $1,254,451,641

Orencia: Abatacept – an injectable used for treating rheumatoid arthritis in adults and juvenile idiopathic arthritis in children – $1,188,411,778

Androgel: Testosterone gel – used to treat a lack of natural testosterone – $1,182,514,119

Nasonex Mometasone furoate – nasal spray for allergy – $1,124,061,350

Tamiflu: Oseltamivir – an antiviral that blocks the actions of influenza virus types A and B

– $1,050,683,805

Vesicare: solifenacin – reduces bladder spasms to treat symptoms of overactive bladder, frequent or urgent urination, and incontinence – $1,040,724,740

Eliquis: Apixaban – a novel anticoagulant – $964,121,283

Cimzia: Certolizumab – injectable for the treatment of rheumatoid arthritis and Crohn's D – $$933,953,154

Namenda XR: Memantine – for moderate to severe Alzheimer's disease – $857,157,299

Levemir: Insulindetemir – long-acting, sub-cutaneous injection insulin for diabetes – $851,149,040

Pradaxa: Dabigatran – a novel anticoagulant – $850,313,699

Prolia: Denosumab – injection for postmenopausal osteoporosis – $817,906,368

Pristiq: Desvenlafaxine – an antidepressant serotonin-norepinephrine reuptake inhibitor – $750,241,124

Nuvaring – a combined hormonal contraceptive vaginal ring – $690,996,076

Zostavax – Shingles vaccine – $686,790,521

Dulera: Mometasone + formoterol – an inhaled medicine to control and prevent asthma – $669,637,717

Gardasil – a human papillomavirus vaccine used to vaccinate against cervical cancer – $659,747,125

Exelon: Rivastigmine – for mild to moderate dementia of the Alzheimer's type and dementia due to Parkinson's disease – $647,136,515

Simponi: Golimumab – helps relieve the pain, stiffness and swelling of moderate to severe rheumatoid arthritis (RA) – $608,898,230

Mirena – a long-acting, reversible birth control hormonal intrauterine device (IUD) – $603,038,710

Onglyza: Saxagliptin – an oral diabetes medicine – $579,325,631

Linzess: Linaclotide – for chronic constipation – $515,749,802

Premarin: Conjugated estrogens – used to treat symptoms of menopause – $493,812,315

Intuniv: Guanfacine – for

attention deficit hyperactivity disorder (ADHD) in children – $489,285,664

Chantix: Varenicline – used to treat nicotine addiction – $472,869,473

Avodart: Dutasteride – used to treat benign prostatic hyperplasia – $471,499,125

Xeljanz: Tofacitinib – for moderate to severe adult Rheumatoid Arthritis – $413,374,592

Uloric: Febuxostat – used to lower blood uric acid levels in adults with gout – $411,824,301

Farxiga: Dapagliflozin – an oral diabetes medicine – $410,997,209

Myrbetriq: Mirabegron – reduces muscle spasms of the bladder and urinary tract – $408,957,063

Premarin Vaginal – conjugated estrogens vaginal cream for post menopausal symptoms – $397,570,841

Epipen 2-Pak: Epinephrine injection – auto-injectors for life-threatening allergic reactions – $389,528,868

Vimovo: Esomeprazole + Naproxen – combination nonsteroidal anti-inflammatory drug – $368,883,419

Epiduo: Adapalene and Benzoyl peroxide – gel combination used to treat acne – $349,457,182

Relpax: Eletriptan – used to treat migraine headaches – $331,629,578

Nexplanon: Etonogestrel implant – small rod inserted under skin for contraception – $301,889,830

Aczone: Dapsone – an anti-infective topical gel used to help treat acne – $278,671,485

Lovaza: Omega 3 fatty acids combination – to reduce triglyceride (TG) levels – $259,812,629

Lipitor: Atorvastatin – a statin used primarily as a lipid-lowering agent – $251,981,518

Axiron: Testosterone – topical solution underarm treatment – $233,871,526

Cymbalta: Duloxetine – for major depressive disorder, general anxiety disorder – $223,291,761

Toviaz: Fesoterodine – used to help treat symptoms of overactive bladder (OAB) –

$219,986,729

Livalo: Pitavastatin – a statin used to improve blood cholesterol levels – $185,479,248

Jublia: Efinaconazole Solution 10% – a topical solution to treat toenail fungus – $178,047,175

Actonel: Rsedronate – a bisphosphonate for preventing and treating osteoporosis – $152,123,935

Breo Ellipta: Luticasone + Vilanterol – a combination inhaled corticosteroid and long-acting beta2-adrenergic agonists to treat chronic obstructive pulmonary disease (COPD) – $140,349,328

Flumist: Quadrivalent Nasal Influenza Vaccine – $131,614,245

Xiaflex: Collagenase clostridium histolyticum – used to treat Dupuytren's contracture – $127,063,110

Quillivant XR: Methylphenidate – for attention deficit hyperactivity disorder (ADHD) – $107,092,690

Belviq Lorcaserin – a weight-loss drug – $96,038,704

Aciphex: Rabeprazole – a PPI for stomach and esophagus problems (acid reflux, ulcer) – $91,853,217

Latisse: Bimatoprost – increases the growth, length, thickness and darkness of eyelashes – $82,671,844

Lunesta: Eszopiclone – a sedative and a hypnotic – $79,894,370

Singulair: Montelukast – used for the maintenance treatment of asthma – $78,256,791

Niaspan: Niacin – used as lipid metabolism regulators – $71,761,121

Estring: estradiol vaginal ring – to relieve moderate to severe itching, burning, and dryness in and around the vagina due to menopause – $71,006,566

Anoro Ellipta: Umeclidinium + Vilanterol – inhalation powder combination to treat COPD – $64,460,164

Plavix: Clopidogrel – an oral antiplatelet anticoagulant – $52,762,015

Botox – $51,501,869

Yaz-28 – estrogen and progestin combination birth control pills – $49,432,035

Osphena: Ospemifene – a selective estrogen receptor modulator (SERM) to relieve pain during sexual intercourse – $49,034,121

Ambien CR: Zolpidem – used for the treatment of insomnia – $45,955,805

Aricept: Donepezil – for mild to moderate dementia caused by Alzheimer's disease – $26,773,067

Brisdelle: Paroxetine – a selective serotonin reuptake inhibitors (SSRIs) antidepressant – $22,581,016

Omnaris: Ciclesonide Nasal Spray – treats seasonal nasal allergy symptoms – $19,352,785

Flomax: Tamsulosi – relaxes muscles, prostate and bladder, making it easier to urinate – $18,139,072

Trilipix: Fenofibrate – a fibrate used to reduce cholesterol levels – $16,459,450

Boniva: Ibandronate – an oral and intravenous bisphosphonate for treating osteoporosis – $16,056,457

Caduet: Amlodipine + Atorvastatin – a combination used to treat high blood pressure or angina that occurs with high cholesterol or triglyceride levels – $14,166,476

Duavee: Conjugated Estrogens and Bazedoxifene – combination product to help reduce and to prevent bone loss (osteoporosis) after menopause – $13,567,296

Reclast: Zoledronic acid – a bisphosphonate for treatment and prevention of postmenopausal osteoporosis and to increase bone mass in men with osteoporosis – $11,208,523

Seasonique: Levonorgestrel, Ethinyl estradiol – a birth control pill – **$11,101,960**

Botox Cosmetic – for moderate to severe frown lines and crow's feet – $952,021

Victoza Unsp N-N: Liraglutide (NN2211) – for obesity

Grand Total

= ***$112,494,804,575***

And I claim most of these illnesses for which these drugs are prescribed are avoidable or preventable

Section 4:

Tests and Diagnoses

27. Early Diagnosis & Treatment

Get It Seen, Get It Diagnosed, Get It Fixed

Meticulous attention to our health provides benefits of which most of us will forever be unaware. This is the paradox of preventive medicine: "What you never had you'll never miss." If the patients don't get ill they ascribe it to their own behavior or even good luck, and while both may play a part, they never make the connection as to good specific preventive medical information or advice. Then again, good preventive medical advice, as explained, has been pretty thin on the ground.

We most often don't notice any of the insidious changes such as high blood pressure or cholesterol that have long-term sequelae. But even if patients follow most of the preventive recommendations, there is another very important facet that I vociferously advocate, and that is getting every minor ailment attended to immediately. Many people are admirable stoics who don't complain about feeling ill, or about what they consider a minor injury, but this oversight is fraught with danger.

Consider the following two animal studies. (I have seen the results confirmed in humans—it's just easier to study animals.)

One was on the Mississippi River, where opossums were threatened with extinction from raccoons and other predators. They suffered scratches, bites, abrasions and even open wounds and, of course, couldn't treat them. The severe wounds became infected and those opossums died, but others with even minor scratches didn't do too well either. They lost weight, their fur fell out, they looked sick and they stopped breeding. This was mainly attributed to stress, and they recovered wonderfully when put on an island where there were no predators. While stress certainly played a big part, also their wounds didn't heal as quickly or as well as they should. Which came first, the chicken or the egg? Did the stress make the wounds and healing worse or did the wounds make the stress worse? Whatever. The point is that these minor afflictions dragged down the overall health of these animals.

The second study is research that showed that mild infections without symptoms of illness can still lead to serious consequences by reducing the lifespan of the infected individuals. The "individuals" in this case were birds, and the infection was thought to speed up the aging process by shortening the telomeres (i.e., the chromosome ends) at a faster rate, thereby accelerating senescence. The researchers note, "Until now, the research community had believed that mild infections that do not produce symptoms of illness have no effect on survival and reproduction.... If this is a general mechanism for any type of mild, chronic infection, which is quite possible, it will mean our study is of major interest to understand the impact that mild illnesses can have on other organisms, including humans." The small, non-measureable effects of the chronic disease appear to underlie the accelerated shortening of the telomeres. When the telomeres get too short, this has a fatal effect and causes premature death.[95]

I have to agree, as for decades I have seen the detrimental effects that minor neglect has had on my patients who chose to ignore or minimize their health care or advice.

To extrapolate this research to human medical experience:

Treat all conditions no matter how minor.

Treat them immediately and get them fully better.

There is a germ, which to the ordinary person is "just a sore throat," but one which can strike fear and dread into the minds of doctors and, literally, the hearts (and kidneys) of the patients. It is clinically impossible to diagnose that it is so "special." Ninety-nine times out of a hundred, indeed it is "just a sore throat." However, this awful germ, identified more accurately as a beta-hemolytic streptococcus (Lancefield Beta Gp 12, from memory), unlike other "strep throats," causes an immune reaction in the patient's hearts and kidneys leading, later in life, to heart valve problems and glomerulonephritis, or the equivalent of kidney shutdown. Some very famous people have had their lives or careers cut short by this germ, including one of the world's richest men, a national leader, a king, a pope and one of the world's greatest footballers and crooners.

Left untreated, glomerulonephritis and rheumatic heart disease can lead to heart or kidney transplants; but beta-hemolytic streptococcus is usually very susceptible to penicillin. Hence the importance of treating, aggressively and immediately, even ostensibly "minor" ailments such as a sore throat or tonsillitis.

"Drug" is not necessarily a dirty word.

In pre-antibiotic days people talked about how little Johnny had a "weak chest." Little Johnny never seemed to be without a cold, and it then developed into a productive cough and then he was coughing up discolored phlegm and was quite ill. Occasionally you still see kids with green nasal discharges and a loose cough you can hear across a busy street. When discolored sputum develops, and it may on top of a viral URTI, it means there is a secondary bacterial infection. Antibiotics are anti-bacterial and now should be prescribed. Like the previous examples of kids with the sore throats that ended up having heart or kidney transplants, their parents either considered it to be a trivial condition or they have been fed misinformation. The child needs antibiotics. But many parents say they don't believe in antibiotics, and there is a worldwide movement to reduce their use. This is informed good medical advice, as too many antibiotics have been used for viral colds which they wont fix, and it causes antibiotic resistance. However, the pressure put on PCP/GPs not to prescribe antibiotics by the government and ivory tower "experts" is questionable in its theoretical approach. Often a stitch in time saves nine. Patients may develop pneumonia or severe bronchitis and need buckets of antibiotics, when prompt treatment would have cleared up the problem much more easily.

Once again I emphasize being a clinician—a doctor who actually has to treat the patient and not hand down "advice" from a government office. If they were serious, as I proposed way back in 1964 as a medical student, they would stop the mega-doses of antibiotics being fed to cattle, chickens and most domestic animals (including salmon and other farmed fish) who are not even ill but are fed these drugs as a preventive. Then there are the many countries where even the most powerful antibiotics can be bought over the counter without a prescription. No wonder there is increasing resistance.

However, without the immediate repair which antibiotic treatment provides, the little Johnnys of yesteryear were often doomed to a long-term burden of chronic problems, and in many cases the result of the so-called `weak chest" was premature death. Antibiotics administered correctly can remove this possibility.

Again, this advice is not meant to endorse the use of antibiotics in viral infections, like the common cold, where they don't work. Be reassured: antibiotics are nothing to be scared of, especially when prescribed by a good clinician. Used wisely, antibiotics are a miracle.

Even with good preventive maintenance there are, unfortunately, many illnesses that we can't avoid despite our best efforts. However, there are also many illnesses that we may think are unavoidable but that can, if diagnosed early, be prevented from developing into something very serious. Regular visits to your GP are an important part of the ***Live Longest*** plan.

Treat all conditions no matter how minor.

Treat them immediately and get them fully better.

Repair activates and optimizes health.

History & Examination

The difference between the ***Live Longest*** check-up and an ordinary annual check-up is that it focuses on those illnesses most likely to affect you and takes into account the age group of the patient.

Some investigation require specialized equipment—eye, mammograms

Examinations of the following systems are recommended.

Preliminary Measurements:

Height and weight, BMI, Waist-hip ratio
Skin – dermoscopy
Cardiovascular
Central nervous system
Respiratory system
Gastro intestinal system
Genito-urinary System: male/female
Endocrine
ENT (Ear, Nose, Throat). Eyes – visual acuity and fields, fundi.
Hearing – auditory acuity
Musculoskeletal/Locomotor
Psychiatric/Mental
Age grip, mobility, posture, nutrition, hydration, feet, walk speed

Medical Symptoms & Signs

The earlier an illness can be diagnosed the more chance of a cure. It is therefore important for you to know what symptoms and signs to look for and not to ignore them. The following is a list of the main signs and symptoms which should be reported.

General

Undue fatigue or tiredness

Unexplained loss of weight

Unexplained bruising / prolonged bleeding

Any blood transfusions

Slowness of movement or mental process

Eyes

Grittiness / inflammation / watering / discharge

Pain & blurring

Loss of vision

Stuck lids

GIT (Gastro Intestinal Tract)

Heartburn/indigestion

Abdominal pain

Change of bowel habit

PR mucus, blood, slime

Weight loss

Yellow whites of eyes

Recurrent diarrhea

Intolerance to bread

CVS (Cardiovascular System)

Blood pressure

Palpitations/fluttering

SOBOE (Shortness of breath on effort)

Chest pain

Swollen ankles

Respiratory

Smoking

Persistent cough / blood in sputum

Wheeze / asthma / difficulty breathing

Bad snoring / choking in sleep

Any previous exposure to asbestos

CNS (Central Nervous System)

KOd

Transient loss of vision / consciousness (TIA)

Altered behavior

Fits

Pins and needles

Weakness of grip

Disturbances of balance

New headache

Tremors

Increasing forgetfulness / confusion

Locomotor / Muscle or joints

Pain

Swelling

Inflammation

Joint pains – note any climbing stairs

Increasing tendency to choke on food

Unaccounted for limp

Finger nodes

Weaker grip

Endocrine

Slowing down (compared with 1 year ago)

Thinning hair

Menstrual problems

Pop eyes

Fast talk

Central obesity

Thirst, polyuria

Work

Exposure to asbestos, diesel, pesticides, sun

Men

Diminished stream & cut off

Frequency/nocturia

Terminal dribbling

Pink urine

Testicular lumps

Women

Any lump

Mammogram/pap

Stress incontinence

Frequency/nocturia

Cystitis/pink urine

Discharge / Inter-menstrual bleeding

Age

Trouble getting out of chairs

Increasingly fixed opinions

Memory problems

Feet – not cared for

Back pain

Mental Health

Feeling something is wrong

Sadness / hopelessness / worthlessness

Worried all the time

Loss of interest

Inappropriate guilt

Sleep difficulties

Suicidal thoughts

Memory problems

Repetition

Tests & Investigations

Medical tests and investigations are important tools in the early diagnosis of potentially life-threatening and/or debilitating illnesses. It is the ***Live Longest*** contention that screening tests must be specific tests focused for your age and sex. When I was a young whippy Medical Registrar I coined the abbreviation "ETK" for all the patients I admitted—it stood for "Every Test Known." As this was an advanced medical unit and I had to find out what others had not, I thought I was pretty smart and at the leading edge of modern medicine.

Oh dear.

Not only was it not cost-effective, it was extremely inefficient. But while I learned my lesson, I still find some colleagues doing the same—ordering ETK in the desperate hope they may find something. I even asked one if he had missed the "Serum Uranium" and he thought I was serious. This is a scattershot approach, when focussed attention to what illness is most likely is preferable.

In 2001, the Director of the Center for Disease Control in Atlanta, USA (the NASA of medicine) declared (with respect to colon cancer): "Screening saves lives... 90% are cured if diagnosed and treated early enough."

"Nine out of ten heart attacks can now be predicted."[96]

"This finding suggests that approaches to prevention can be based on similar principles and have the potential to prevent most premature cases of myocardial infarction."[97]

The challenge is to select those tests that are cost-effective. They should give an answer as to where a cure or improvement can be made, given your age. It is important that both the patient and physician realize the necessity, desirability and usefulness of all investigations and any risks involved (such as with CT scans).

What Tests Should Be Done

Live Longest has been very careful to select the best and correct *clinical* evidence, tests and treatments based on the experience of practicing clinical consultants. There is a battery of tests appropriate for each age group and sex. "Common things occur most commonly"—so it is most important (at least six times as important) to screen your cardiac risks. Rare or expensive tests should only be done if your history and examination suggests they are necessary or if you wish to pay for it to satisfy your curiosity or anxiety. The basic tests that follow do not carry any significant risks. If you do need further complex tests, then any risks should be fully explained.

ECG/EKGs and stress testing have long been considered by many cardiologists as part of CVS screening. But are they predictive and cost-effective? Probably not. Would you have them done? Probably yes.

Some screening tests such as mammography and pap smears have been introduced as "recommended" but debate has raged as to cost-effectiveness and restrictions have been invariably imposed to attract a rebate.

Meanwhile a FBC (Full Blood Count) and MBA (Multiple Biochemical Analysis) are so ubiquitous that they are accepted as "necessary" when often they are not.

Medicine often gets caught trying to be all things to all people. However, the following tests and investigations are considered to be both cost-effective and evidenced. These should be undertaken on the judgement of the clinician. Any abnormalities progress to secondary tests.

A recent study concluded that screening is overused for some diseases and possibly it is perceived as more effective and cost-effective than it is. The role of screening should be considered on a disease-specific basis. Of 39 screening tests for 19 diseases, screening was only recommended for 6 of them and does not result in reductions in all-cause mortality. Disease-specific mortality was reduced between 16% and 45% for only 4 screening tests: ultrasound for abdominal aortic aneurysm in men; mammography for breast cancer; and fecal occult blood test and flexible sigmoidoscopy for colorectal cancer. Additional screening tests associated with reduced disease-specific mortality in individual trials included visual inspection for cervical cancer, alpha-fetoprotein and ultrasound for hepatocellular cancer, and visual examination for oral cancer.[98]

As stated previously, I agree, and recommend investigations, not only on a "disease-specific basis," but uniquely, also on an age- and sex-specific basis.

Recommended Age-Specific Tests Selected From:

Blood and biochemical FBC/ESR/CRP, MBA including Blood Glucose

Cardiovascular check – Cholesterol HDL:LDL, Triglycerides, ECG/EKG annually over 65

Prostate check

Gynecology check – Pap, Mammogram, DEXA

Colon cancer check – Colonoscopy (age 50 or 40 if smoking, drinking, male)

Skin check – dermoscopy

Coeliac D – IgA TTG and serum IgA

Metabolic and others – as indicated from history and examination

Chest x-ray (PA & lateral)

What These Tests Are and What They Are For

1. Hematology: FBC = Full Blood Count

Hemoglobin – indicates if you are anemic

White Cell Count – indicates infection, leukemia

ESR – indicates inflammation

Platelet Count – indicates bleeding problems

CRP – indicates inflammation

2. Biochemistry: MBA = Multiple Biochemical Analysis

Sodium, potassium, chloride, bicarbonate, anion gap, osmolality are the electrolytes which compose the body fluids & their balance

Calcium/Phosphate/Alkaline phosphatase – bone disorders

Urea & Creatinine – indicate kidney function

Urate – elevated in gout & metabolic syndrome in children & adolescents[99]

Glucose – elevated in Diabetes

Protein (Albumin and Globulin) – low in kidney and some liver disease and high in some metabolic disorders (Myeloma)

Bilirubin – indicates gall bladder/liver disease

The "ase(s)" are enzymes which indicate liver and sometimes heart problems

Iron – low in blood loss – from piles to cancer

3. Lipids

Cholesterol – subdivided into good HDL and bad LDL; elevated LDL considered a major heart risk

Triglycerides – one of the lipids – elevation considered a heart risk

4. Coeliac Disease Antibodies – see section on Coeliac Disease, sequel book.

5. Colonoscopy/Endoscopy

A camera on the end of a photo-optic cable is inserted via the anus to examine the lower gut. Patients are mostly sedated and the actual procedure is painless. It can detect Cancer of the Colon (CAC) early enough to effect a cure. FOBT (Fecal Occult Blood Tests) are blotting paper tests on your feces for minute amounts of blood. They are cheaper, less embarrassing but not as good. Colonoscopy is "The Gold Standard."

Endoscopes are passed via the mouth into the stomach to look for ulcers or cancers.

6. Other specific tests as indicated (e.g., Thyroid Function)

7. ECG/EKG: Detects any abnormalities of heart rhythm and rate at rest and evidence of any old infarcts.

8. Cardiac Stress Test

This determines any sinister changes with exercise and if okay, indicates that exercise does not provoke dangerous changes.

9. Coronary Scoring

Detects any calcium in coronary arteries, which is one indicator of degenerative disease. It is of some 51% help with respect to predicting acute cardiac events (heart attacks); that is, it is not the full answer. However, it further helps provide more information about the most important aspect of our health (our heart).

10. PSA – Prostate-Specific Antigen

Indicates either prostate enlargement—Benign Prostatic Enlargement (BPH)—or cancer.

PSA presents an ethical problem in that, if it is elevated, it is not diagnostic; so you are then faced with the dilemma, according to your age, as to what to do. You can investigate further and if it is cancer, have treatment which often leads to impotence and incontinence; or, let it go, as it is very slow growing, and the average duration of life if untreated is another 10 years. Thus if you are 50 you have a decision; but if you are 70 maybe not. According to the above philosophy, if you get it done, you may choose to repeat it every 5 years or so. The one laboratory keeps a comparative record which is preferable to having it done elsewhere.

11. DEXA

This is a special x-ray to detect osteoporosis. Heel-bone densities are not satisfactory.

12. Dermoscopy

These are hand-held or cable-optic cameras that optically take away the top layer of skin so the examiner can see better the histology of the mole or skin lesion underneath; it enhances the diagnosis of melanoma and skin cancers.

Age-Specific Tests

Normal Values

The United States reports many values in mg/liter, where the United Kingdom, Europe, Australia and New Zealand use mom/l. All laboratories give their normal range after the test specimen results.

Normal values may differ slightly between laboratories. Slight abnormalities need interpretation by a doctor, but usually a repeat test can be done after a suitable interval to see if the abnormality persists.

The following table provides a quick checklist of suggested recommended tests according to age group and gender.

This table of tests is only a guide and represents screening at a first attendance.

Some tests may not need to be repeated. After a baseline around 20 years, lipids should be done every 5 years.[100]

10-year screening otherwise is suggested, reducing to 5-year intervals after 45 years or as clinically assessed.

AGE	MALE	FEMALE
15-30	CXR (PA & lateral) FBC/ESR/CRP, MBA Coeliac D Cardiovascular check Others as indicated STD (4% asymptomatic)	CXR (PA & lateral) FBC/ESR/CRP, MBA Coeliac D Cardiovascular check Gynecology (Pap, breasts, STD) Others as indicated
30-40	CXR (PA & lateral) FBC/ESR/CRP, MBA Coeliac D Cardiovascular check incl. LDL Others as indicated	CXR (PA & lateral) FBC/ESR/CRP, MBA Coeliac D Cardiovascular check incl. LDL Gynecology – Pap smear, breasts Others as indicated
40-50	CXR (PA & lateral) FBC/ESR/CRP, MBA Coeliac D Cardiovascular check Prostrate check Colon Cancer Others as indicated	CXR (PA & lateral) FBC/ESR/CRP, MBA Coeliac D Cardiovascular check Gynecology (Pap, mammogram, DEXA) Colon Cancer Others as indicated
50–64	CXR (PA & lateral) FBC/ESR/CRP, MBA Coeliac D Cardiovascular check Prostrate check Colon Cancer Others as indicated Hearing	CXR (PA & lateral) FBC/ESR/CRP, MBA Coeliac D Cardiovascular check Gynecology Colon Cancer Others as indicated Vision
65–74	ECG/EKG annual – exclude AF Ultrasonography for Abdominal Aortic Aneurysm	ECG/EKG annually – exclude AF

High-Value Cancer Screening: American College of Physicians Recommendations

This section gives practicing clinicians a quick reference for evidence-based recommendations on cancer screening in asymptomatic, average-risk adults.

Breast: For women aged 40–49 years, mammography screening every 2 years should be offered if a woman requests it after a discussion of the potential benefits and harms. For women aged 50–74 years who are in good health, mammography should be encouraged every 2 years.

Cervical Cancer is perceived as a disease of young women, but more older women die from it than younger ones. Pap smears should be done until age 70 at least.[101] For women aged 21–29 years, cytology testing is recommended every 3 years. For those aged 30–65, cytology plus HPV testing can be done every 5 years (instead of cytology alone).

The 9-valent human papillomavirus vaccine can potentially prevent 80% of cervical cancers if given to all 11- or 12-year-old children before they are exposed to the virus. The study also found the 9-valent vaccine, under the trademark of Gardasil-9, has the potential to protect against an additional 8% of oropharyngeal cancers, which include the base of the tongue and tonsils. This disease is the second most common HPV-associated cancer.[102]

Ovarian: Screening isn't recommended.

Colorectal: For patients aged 50–75 years, one of the following strategies should be encouraged: high-sensitivity fecal occult blood testing (FOBT) or fecal immunofluorescence testing (FIT) annually; sigmoidoscopy every 5 years; combined high-sensitivity FOBT or FIT every 3 years plus sigmoidoscopy every 5 years; or optical colonoscopy every 10 years.

Using data from a meta-analysis of randomized controlled trials, it was concluded that reductions in cancer-specific mortality take about a decade to become apparent, so less screening, or none at all, might be better in people with limited life expectancy. In a linked editorial, however, it was argued that this conclusion rests on the "questionable assumption" that absolute improvements in colorectal cancer mortality in older adults are similar to those in middle-aged adults;[103] in fact, the risk of such mortality increases sharply in older age, with a corresponding increase in the benefits of screening. The time to benefit from screening "might be substantially shorter" than the study estimates, especially for adults who have not previously been screened. So less screening is not necessarily better.

Prostate: For men aged 50–69 with a life expectancy of at least a decade, discuss screening's benefits and risks. If patients prefer screening, do prostate-specific antigen testing once every 2–4 years.

Aortic Aneurysm

Males, especially smokers > 65 years, should have an abdominal ultrasound. Abdominal aneurysms are found in 4 to 8%, but 43% reduction in fatal ruptures is possible.

Young Athletes

- Have a 2.5 higher risk of sudden death. Should have a full CVS screen (history, exam & ECG/EKG) every 2 years from 12 years old.
- Could cut heart deaths by 50–70%, especially for HCM (Hypertrophic Cardiomyopathy).

Unnecessary ECGs/EKGs

Asymptomatic adults at low risk for developing cardiovascular disease do not benefit from cardiac screening with electrocardiography, stress electrocardiography, or myocardial perfusion imaging.[104]

Statins boost survival rate of cancer by up to 47%.[105]

In a 14-year follow up of people being treated with statins for high cholesterol, it was found statins were associated with reduced mortality and improved survival in the four most common cancers, with lower risk of death in lung, breast, prostate and bowel cancers:
prostate: 47% lower risk of death (5 year survival rates)
breast: 43%
bowel: 30%
lung: 22%

Epilogue

To actually show the surgery I perform, here is Onelia, who at age 90 was 15 years older than I was, at 75 years, when a colleague in my clinic diagnosed a cancer on her nose (the dotted outline) and referred her to a University Teaching Hospital. They put her on the back burner (waiting list) as, according to her, they didn't want to do it; my colleague never received any feedback from the hospital.

Onelia, whom I had previously looked after, then issued her ultimatum that either I do it or she wouldn't get it done. I did it and didn't charge her. Perhaps I am wrong but I'm pretty sure that, had she been operated on in hospital, she would have had a general anaesthetic and an ugly graft slapped on. I hate grafts on noses, as the nose is the most obvious part of our appearance; grafts are invariably hideous, and patients are forever self-conscious. Heart in mouth, and using local anaesthesia, this is the operation I did. Her smiley face some six weeks later says it all:

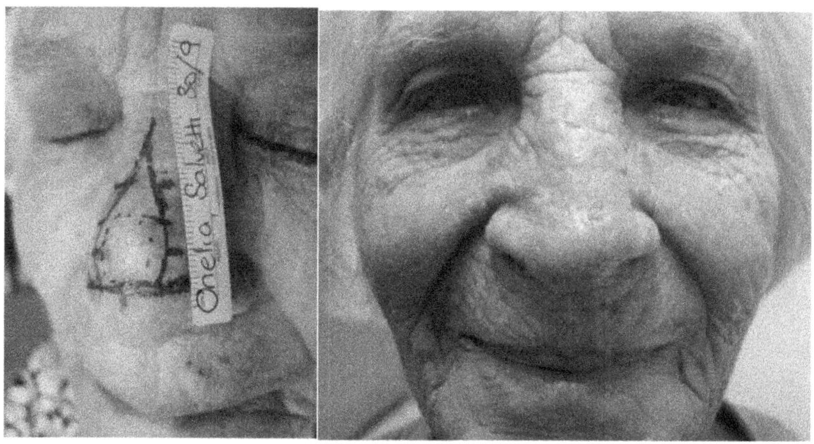

P.S. Onelia is Italian and worked physically hard on a farm all her life (growing tobacco). When I gave her my "Newtrition" diet she tolerantly explained to me that it is what she had been eating all her life. My Newtrition is based on the Mediterranean (Italian) diet. She also walks everywhere, is lean, lives alone and looks after herself. No wonder she is spry and with it at 90—but I could and did add a few "improvements" for her, as I feel "it's never too late"—in contrast to the hospital's unvoiced attitude. I regarded her operation, even if she was 90, as not only desirable but essential. A year later, she feels confident about her looks, is alive and kicking, bopping and shopping and not dying of cancer in some nursing home.

She paid me more than I dared hope for when I thanked her for allowing me use these photos. She grasped me and looked into my eyes and said "No, thank *you!*"

That's the best reward a doctor ever gets.

Endnotes

1. Editorial annals of Internal Medicine 1999.
2. Ann Int Med 2003:139 Supplement.
3. Ritual, Not Science, Keeps the Annual Physical Alive. *Medscape*. Apr 06, 2015.
4. General health checks in adults for reducing morbidity and mortality from disease. Cochrane Database Syst Rev. 2012 Oct 17;10:CD009009.
5. Ritual, Not Science, Keeps the Annual Physical Alive. *Medscape*. Apr 06, 2015.
6. Ward BW, Black LI. State and Regional Prevalence of Diagnosed Multiple Chronic Conditions Among Adults Aged ≥ 18 Years—United States, 2014. MMWR Morb Mortal Wkly Rep 2016;65:735–738. doi:\
7. http://dx.doi.org/10.15585/mmwr.mm6529a3.
8. Br Heart J. 1987 Jun; 57(6): 497–502. PMCID: PMC1277217. The history of coronary care units.
9. Cardiosource, 27 Mar 2007.
10. Center for Disease Control and Prevention (CDC) and *New Yorker*, "A Bug In The System," 26 Jan 2015.
11. Pimentel M, Morales W, Rezaie A, et al. Development and Validation of a Biomarker for Diarrhea-Predominant Irritable Bowel Syndrome in Human Subjects. PLOS ONE. 2015.
12. Malins J. Fence or ambulance? Bulletin of the North Carolina State Board of Health 1913;27(10):16. Available at:
13. http://www.archive.org/stream/bulletinofnorthc27nort# page/16/mode/1up
14. University of East Anglia. "Could a computer tell you when your time is up?" ScienceDaily. 30 March 2016.
15. <www.sciencedaily.com/releases/2016/03/160330211029.htm>.
16. http://www.foodbusinessnews.net/articles/news_home /Business_News/2014/11/Aging_gracefully.aspx?ID =%7B44E938EE-973C-4EB4-AF02-378C30C49141%7D&cck=1
17. WHO 2004.
18. Steven N. Austad, Kathleen E. Fischer. Sex Differences in Lifespan. *Cell Metabolism*, 2016; 23 (6): 1022. doi: 10.1016/j.cmet.2016.05.019
19. Hiram Beltrán-Sánchez, Caleb E. Finch, Eileen M. Crimmins. Twentieth century surge of excess adult male mortality. *Proceedings of the National Academy of Sciences*, 2015; 201421942. doi: 10.1073/pnas.1421942112

20. Steven N. Austad, Kathleen E. Fischer. Sex Differences in Lifespan. *Cell Metabolism*, 2016; 23 (6): 1022. doi: 10.1016/j.cmet.2016.05.019
21. Ohio State University, *Journal of Occupational and Environmental Health*, June 2016.
22. Impact of a 6-wk olive oil supplementation in healthy adults on urinary proteomic biomarkers of coronary artery disease, chronic kidney disease, and diabetes (types 1 and 2): a randomized, parallel, controlled, double-blind study. Sandra Silva, Maria R Bronze, Maria E Figueira, Justina Siwy, Harald Mischak, Emilie Combet, and William Mullen. First published November 19, 2014. doi: 10.3945/ ajcn.114.094219. Am J Clin Nutr ajcn.094219.
23. Aging Cell. 2015 Aug; 14(4): 497–510. Published online 2015 Apr 22. doi: 10.1111/acel.12338 PMCID: PMC4531065 Interventions to Slow Aging in Humans: Are We Ready?
24. published online April 11 in JAMA.
25. The Association Between Income and Life Expectancy in the United States, 2001-2014 Raj Chetty, PhD; Michael Stepner, BA; Sarah Abraham, BA; Shelby Lin, MPhil; Benjamin Scuderi, BA; Nicholas Turner, PhD; Augustin Bergeron, MA; David Cutler, PhD4*JAMA*. Published online April 10, 2016. doi:10.1001/jama.2016.4226
26. Office for National Statistics, UK, 2016.
27. Emanuel EJ. Why I hope to die at 75. *Atlantic,* 2014 Oct. www.theatlantic.com/features/archive/2014/09 /why-i-hope-to-die-at-75/379329/.
28. Harvard University. “Longer life, disability free: Increases in life expectancy accompanied by increase in disability-free life expectancy, study shows.” ScienceDaily, 6 June 2016. <www.sciencedaily.com/releases/2016/06/160606120039.htm>.
29. The paper is titled “Understanding the Improvement in Disability Free Life Expectancy in the U.S. Elderly Population,” NBER Working Paper No. 22306.
30. *BMJ* 2015; 350:h292.
31. The Okinawa (Program) Way by B.Wilcox, C. Wilcox and M. Suzuki. Publisher: Clarkson Potter 2001, then Michael Joseph and Penguin.
32. The Global BMI Mortality Collaboration. Body-mass index and all-cause mortality: individual-participant-data meta-analysis of 239 prospective studies in four continents. *The Lancet*, 2016. doi: 10.1016/S0140-6736(16)30175-1
33. Berkley Earth, August 2015 (accepted for publication in PLOS One).

34. Turner, Erick H. et al., Selective Publication of Antidepressant Trials and Its Influence on Apparent Efficacy, *New England Journal of Medicine*, 17 January 2008; 252–60.
35. *J Intern Med.* Published online March 16, 2016.
36. *MMWR* surveillance summary.
37. American Academy of Neurology news release April 2016.
38. International Journal of Epidemiology online report January 15, 2015.
39. *BMJ* 2012; 345:e5568. doi: http://dx.doi.org/10.1136/bmj.e5568 (Published 30 August 2012).
40. *New York Times.*
41. *BMJ*, 2016; i1209. doi: 10.1136/bmj.i1209
42. M. Guzman-Castillo, R. Ahmed, N. Hawkins, S. Scholes, E. Wilkinson, J. Lucy, S. Capewell, M. O'Flaherty, R. Raine, M. Bajekal. The contribution of primary prevention medication and dietary change in coronary mortality reduction in England between 2000 and 2007: a modelling study. *BMJ Open*, 2015; 5 (1): e006070. doi: 10.1136/bmjopen-2014-006070
43. Medical error—the third leading cause of death in the US. *BMJ* 2016; 353:i2139. doi: http://dx.doi.org/10.1136/bmj.i2139 (Published 03 May 2016)
44. March 15, 2016 Medscape Internal Medicine.
45. Dima M. Qato, Jocelyn Wilder, L. Philip Schumm, Victoria Gillet, G. Caleb Alexander. Changes in Prescription and Over-the-Counter Medication and Dietary Supplement Use Among Older Adults in the United States, 2005 vs 2011. *JAMA Internal Medicine*, 2016. doi: 10.1001/jamainternmed.2015.8581
46. Drugs & Aging, February 2015, Volume 32, Issue 2, pp 159-167. First online: 08 January 2015. Impact of Multiple Low-Level Anticholinergic Medications on Anticholinergic Load of Community-Dwelling Elderly With and Without Dementia. Karen E. Mate , Karen P. Kerr, Dimity Pond, Evan J.Williams, John Marley, Peter Disler, Henry Brodaty, Parker J. Magin.
47. The Mayo Clinic, January 20, 2016.
48. Christopher T. Ford, Siân Richardson, Francis McArdle, Silvina B. Lotito, Alan Crozier, Anne McArdle, Malcolm J. Jackson. Identification of (poly)phenol treatments that modulate the release of pro-inflammatory cytokines by human lymphocytes. *British Journal of Nutrition*, 2016; 115 (10): 1699. doi: 10.1017/S0007114516000805
49. Simin Nikbin Meydani, D.V.M., Ph.D. et al. Long-term calorie restriction inhibits inflammation without impairing cell-mediated

immunity: A randomized controlled trial in non-obese humans. *Aging*, July 2016.

50. bmjopen June 2016, Volume 6, Number 6. An inverse association between low-density-lipoprotein cholesterol and mortality in the elderly.
51. June 29 in *PLoS One.*
52. July 5 in JAMA Internal Medicine.
53. Martin J O'Donnell, PhD et al. Global and regional effects of potentially modifiable risk factors associated with acute stroke in 32 countries (INTERSTROKE): a case-control study. *The Lancet*, July 2016; doi: 10.1016/S0140-6736(16)30506-2
54. Christopher Murray et al. Global, regional, and national disability-adjusted life years (DALYs) for 306 diseases and injuries and healthy life expectancy (HALE) for 188 countries, 1990-2013: quantifying the epidemiological transition. *The Lancet* 2015; 386 (10009), pp. 2145–2191.
55. LANCET, the Global Burden of Disease Study 2013. Published: June 8, 2015
56. Published in the Proceedings of the National Academy of Sciences 2016.
57. NCHS data brief.
58. 2016 June 30 *National Vital Statistics Reports.*
59. Elsevier Health Sciences. "Americans are getting heart-healthier: Coronary heart disease decreasing in the US: Significant improvements seen across multiple sociodemographic groups." ScienceDaily. ScienceDaily, 15 June 2016. <www.sciencedaily.com/releases/2016/06/160615100358.htm>
60. Thomas A. Dingus, Feng Guo, Suzie Lee, Jonathan F. Antin, Miguel Perez, Mindy Buchanan-King, and Jonathan Hankey. Driver crash risk factors and prevalence evaluation using naturalistic driving data. *PNAS*, February 22, 2016. doi: 10.1073/pnas.1513271113
61. Harding MC, Sloan CD, Merrill RM, et al. Transition from cardiovascular disease to cancer as the leading cause of death in US States, 1999–2013. American Heart Association (AHA) Epidemiology and Prevention and Lifestyle and Cardiometabolic Health (EPI/Lifestyle) 2016 Scientific Sessions; March 3, 2016; Phoenix, AZ.
62. Ford ES, Ajani UA, Croft JB, et al. Explaining the decrease in US deaths from coronary disease, 1980–2000. *N Engl J Med* 2007; 356:2388-2398.

63. Steve Horvath, Michael Gurven, Morgan E. Levine, Benjamin C. Trumble, Hillard Kaplan, Hooman Allayee, Beate R. Ritz, Brian Chen, Ake T. Lu, Tammy M. Rickabaugh, Beth D. Jamieson, Dianjianyi Sun, Shengxu Li, Wei Chen, Lluis Quintana-Murci, Maud Fagny, Michael S. Kobor, Philip S. Tsao, Alexander P. Reiner, Kerstin L. Edlefsen, Devin Absher, Themistocles L. Assimes. An epigenetic clock analysis of race/ethnicity, sex, and coronary heart disease. *Genome Biology*, 2016; 17 (1) DOI: 10.1186/s13059-016-1030-0.
64. Douglas G. Manuel, Richard Perez, Claudia Sanmartin, Monica Taljaard, Deirdre Hennessy, Kumanan Wilson, Peter Tanuseputro, Heather Manson, Carol Bennett, Meltem Tuna, Stacey Fisher, Laura C. Rosella. Measuring Burden of Unhealthy Behaviours Using a Multivariable Predictive Approach: Life Expectancy Lost in Canada Attributable to Smoking, Alcohol, Physical Inactivity, and Diet. *PLOS Medicine*, 2016; 13 (8): e1002082 DOI: 10.1371/journal.pmed.1002082.
65. Ann Int Med 2003:139 Supplement.
66. American Sociological Association. "Relationships with family members, but not friends, decrease likelihood of death." ScienceDaily. ScienceDaily, 21 August 2016. <www.sciencedaily.com/releases/2016/08/160821093058.htm>.
67. David J. Sharrow, James J. Anderson. A Twin Protection Effect? Explaining Twin Survival Advantages with a Two-Process Mortality Model. *PLOS ONE*, 2016; 11 (5): e0154774 DOI: 10.1371/journal.pone.0154774.
68. Murray CJL, Vos T et al. Global, regional, and national incidence, prevalence, and years lived with disability for 301 acute and chronic diseases and injuries in 188 countries, 1990–2013: a systematic analysis for the Global Burden of Disease Study 2013. *The Lancet*, June 2015. doi: 10.1016/S0140-6736(15)60692-4
69. Global Burden of Disease Study 2013 Collaborators. Global, regional, and national incidence, prevalence, and years lived with disability for 301 acute and chronic diseases and injuries in 188 countries, 1990–2013: a systematic analysis for the Global Burden of Disease Study 2013. *The Lancet*, 2015. doi: 10.1016/S0140-6736(15)60692-4
70. Eileen M. Crimmins, Yuan Zhang, Yasuhiko Saito. Trends Over 4 Decades in Disability-Free Life Expectancy in the United States. *American Journal of Public Health*, 2016. doi: 10.2105/AJPH.2016.303120
71. Harvard University. "Longer life, disability free: Increases in life expectancy accompanied by increase in disability-free life expectancy,

study shows." ScienceDaily. ScienceDaily, 6 June 2016. <www.sciencedaily.com/releases/2016/06/160606120039.htm>.

72. JAMA Internal Medicine 2016; online.
73. Morbidity and Mortality Weekly Report 65(29):735–738. Centers for Disease Control and Prevention (CDC), 2016.
74. Lara B. McKenzie, Erica Fletcher, Nicolas G. Nelson, Kristin J. Roberts, Elizabeth G. Klein. Epidemiology of skateboarding-related injuries sustained by children and adolescents 5–19 years of age and treated in US emergency departments: 1990 through 2008. *Injury Epidemiology*, 2016; 3 (1). doi: 10.1186/s40621-016-0075-6
75. Morbidity and Mortality Weekly Report May1, 2009, Vol.58, No.16
76. American College of Cardiology. "Heart attack patients getting younger, more obese: Analysis of 2 decades reveals risk factors are on the rise, despite greater awareness." ScienceDaily. ScienceDaily, 24 March 2016. <www.sciencedaily.com/releases/2016/03/160324192426.htm>.
77. Harding MC, Sloan CD, Merrill RM, et al. Transition from cardiovascular disease to cancer as the leading cause of death in US States, 1999–2013. American Heart Association (AHA) Epidemiology and Prevention and Lifestyle and Cardiometabolic Health (EPI/Lifestyle) 2016 Scientific Sessions; March 3, 2016; Phoenix, AZ. Abstract MP67.
78. Ford ES, Ajani UA, Croft JB, et al. Explaining the decrease in US deaths from coronary disease, 1980–2000. *N Engl J Med* 2007; 356:2388-2398.
79. *JAMA Oncol.* doi:10.1001/jamaoncol.2015.6396.
80. *Ann Fam Med.* 2015;13:472-474. Full text.
81. Dima M. Qato, Jocelyn Wilder, L. Philip Schumm, Victoria Gillet, G. Caleb Alexander. Changes in Prescription and Over-the-Counter Medication and Dietary Supplement Use Among Older Adults in the United States, 2005 vs 2011. *JAMA Internal Medicine*, 2016. doi: 10.1001/jamainternmed.2015.8581
82. Duke Health. "Physical declines begin earlier than expected among U.S. adults." ScienceDaily. ScienceDaily, 21 July 2016. <www.sciencedaily.com/releases/2016/07/160721144805.htm>.
83. Judy R. Dubno, PhD et al. Higher Health Care Costs in Middle-aged US Adults With Hearing Loss. *JAMA Otolaryngology-Head & Neck Surgery*, April 2016. doi: 10.1001/jamaoto.2016.0188
84. *JAMA Otolaryngology—Head & Neck Surgery* article (free).

85. Harvard University. "Longer life, disability free: Increases in life expectancy accompanied by increase in disability-free life expectancy, study shows." ScienceDaily. ScienceDaily, 6 June 2016. <www.sciencedaily.com/releases/2016/06/160606120039.htm>.
86. The Lancet. "'Aging well" must be a global priority, experts say." ScienceDaily. ScienceDaily, 5 November 2014. <www.sciencedaily.com/releases/2014/11/141105203421.htm>
87. Heart Disease and Lifestyle: Why Are Doctors in Denial? *Medscape*. Jan 12, 2015.
88. Robert Mai and Stefan Hoffmann. How to Combat the Unhealthy = Tasty Intuition: The Influencing Role of Health Consciousness. *Journal of Public Policy & Marketing*, January 2015.
89. Henry Ehas, *The Australian*, 27 July 2015.
90. Professor Rodney Daniel Sinclair, Evidence Given to the House of Representatives Standing Committee on Health and Ageing, 43rd Parliament, Official Committee Hansard, Canberra, 21 June 2013, p. 10.
91. Timothy Hoff Practice Under Pressure, Rutgers University Press, 2009.
92. Robert M. Wachter. *New York Times* 18/01/16.
93. Fast Food Nation by Eric Schlosser, Houghton Mifflin Co, 2001, Penguin 2002.
94. *SALT – A WORLD HISTORY*, by Kurlansky, Jonathen Cape, 2002.
95. The Australian 15/01/15.
96. Khadija Ismail, Lisa Nussbaum, Paola Sebastiani, Stacy Andersen, Thomas Perls, Nir Barzilai, Sofiya Milman. Compression of Morbidity Is Observed Across Cohorts with Exceptional Longevity. *Journal of the American Geriatrics Society*, 2016. doi: 10.1111/jgs.14222
97. Paul D. Loprinzi, Adam Branscum, June Hanks, Ellen Smit. Healthy Lifestyle Characteristics and Their Joint Association With Cardiovascular Disease Biomarkers in US Adults. *Mayo Clinic Proceedings*, 2016. doi: 10.1016/j.mayocp.2016.01.009
98. M. Asghar, D. Hasselquist, B. Hansson, P. Zehtindjiev, H. Westerdahl, S. Bensch. Hidden costs of infection: Chronic malaria accelerates telomere degradation and senescence in wild birds. *Science*, 2015; 347 (6220): 436. doi: 10.1126/science.1261121
99. *British Medical Journal 2004;329:527.*
100. *Lancet 2004;364:9437.*
101. Screening Asymptomatic Adults for Disease Does Not Save Lives. International Journal of Epidemiology, online report January 15, 2015.
102. Circ 2207;115:2526-32.

103. Editorial JAMA 2000; 284.
104. Cancer Research UK. Cervical cancer mortality statistics. 2014. www.cancerresearchuk.org/cancer-info/cancerstats/types/cervix/mortality. Elit L. Role of cervical screening in older women. *Maturitas*2014;79:413-20.
105. M. Saraiya, E. R. Unger, T. D. Thompson, C. F. Lynch, B. Y. Hernandez, C. W. Lyu, M. Steinau, M. Watson, E. J. Wilkinson, C. Hopenhayn, G. Copeland, W. Cozen, E. S. Peters, Y. Huang, M. S. Saber, S. Altekruse, M. T. Goodman. US Assessment of HPV Types in Cancers: Implications for Current and 9-Valent HPV Vaccines. *JNCI Journal of the National Cancer Institute*, 2015; 107 (6): djv086. doi: 10.1093/jnci/djv086
106. doi: 10.1136/bmj.h2029
107. Annals of Internal Medicine Source Reference: Chou R, et al. "Cardiac screening with electrocardiography, stress echocardiography, or myocardial perfusion imaging: high-value care advice from the high value care task force of the American College of Physicians" Ann Inter Med 2015. doi: 10.7236/M14-1225.
108. European Society of Cardiology. "Statins may be associated with reduced mortality in 4 common cancers: High cholesterol diagnosis associated with lower risk of death in lung, breast, prostate and bowel cancers." ScienceDaily. ScienceDaily, 8 July 2016. <www.sciencedaily.com/releases/2016/07/160708123619.htm>.
109. Med Sci Sports Exerc. 2007; 39:1401-7

www.ingramcontent.com/pod-product-compliance
Lightning Source LLC
Chambersburg PA
CBHW060030030426
42334CB00019B/2255
* 9 7 8 0 9 9 5 3 9 9 6 1 7 *